ATHLETIC TRAINING CLINICAL EDUCATION GUIDE

ATHLETIC TRAINING CLINICAL EDUCATION GUIDE

Tim Laurent, EdD, ATC, VATL
Lynchburg College, Lynchburg, Virginia

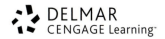

Australia • Brazil • Japan • Korea • Mexico • Singapore • Spain • United Kingdom • United States

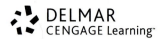

Athletic Training Clinical Education Guide
By Tim Laurent

Vice President, Career and Professional
Editorial: Dave Garza

Director of Learning Solutions: Matthew Kane

Acquisitions Editor: Matt Seeley

Managing Editor: Marah Bellegarde

Senior Product Manager: Darcy M. Scelsi

Editorial Assistant: Samantha Zullo

Vice President, Career and Professional
Marketing: Jennifer McAvey

Marketing Manager: Kristin McNary

Marketing Coordinator: Erica Ropitsky

Production Director: Carolyn Miller

Art Director: Jack Pendleton

Production Technology Analyst:
Mary Colleen Liburdi

For product information and technology assistance, contact us at
Professional & Career Group Customer Support, 1-800-648-7450

For permission to use material from this text or product,
submit all requests online at **cengage.com/permissions.**
Further permissions questions can be e-mailed to
permissionrequest@cengage.com.

Library of Congress Control Number: 2008942908

ISBN-13: 978-1-4354-5360-9

ISBN-10: 1-4354-5360-3

Delmar
5 Maxwell Drive
Clifton Park, NY 12065-2919
USA

Cengage Learning products are represented in Canada by Nelson Education, Ltd.

For your lifelong learning solutions, visit **delmar.cengage.com**

Visit our corporate website at **cengage.com.**

Notice to the Reader
Publisher does not warrant or guarantee any of the products described herein or perform any independent analysis in connection with any of the product information contained herein. Publisher does not assume, and expressly disclaims, any obligation to obtain and include information other than that provided to it by the manufacturer. The reader is expressly warned to consider and adopt all safety precautions that might be indicated by the activities described herein and to avoid all potential hazards. By following the instructions contained herein, the reader willingly assumes all risks in connection with such instructions. The publisher makes no representations or warranties of any kind, including but not limited to, the warranties of fitness for particular purpose or merchantability, nor are any such representations implied with respect to the material set forth herein, and the publisher takes no responsibility with respect to such material. The publisher shall not be liable for any special, consequential, or exemplary damages resulting, in whole or part, from the readers' use of, or reliance upon, this material.

Printed in Canada
1 2 3 4 5 6 7 13 12 11 10 09

CONTENTS

SECTION 4 **Scoring Rubrics**   **247**

Skill Charts

Scoring Rubric	LOT Verification Chart	Novice	Advanced
Vital Signs	42	248	249
Body Composition	43	250	251
Baseline Measurements	44	252	253
Splinting	45	254	255
Equipment Fitting	46	256	257
Taping	47	258	259
Elastic Wraps	48	260	261
Hydration Assessment	49	262	263
Otoscope	57	264	265
Ophthalmoscope	57	264	265
Stethoscope	57	264	265
Foot, Ankle, and Leg Evaluation	66	266	268
Knee, and Thigh Evaluation	68	269	271
Hip Evaluation	70	272	274
Back and Neck Evaluation	72	275	277
Shoulder and Arm Evaluation	74	278	281
Elbow, Wrist, and Hand Evaluation	76	282	284
Head and Face Evaluation	78	285	287
Peak Flow Meter	87	288	289
Body Temperature	87	288	289
Pupil Reaction	87	288	289
Urinalysis	87	288	289
Abdominal Palpation	87	288	289
Throat/neck Palpation	87	288	289
Emergency Management	98	290	291
Patient Transport	98	290	291
Open Wound treatment	98	290	291
Control Bleeding	98	290	291
Immobilization	99	292	293
Crutch Fitting	99	292	293
Modality Application	108	294	296
Therapeutic Exercise – Foot, Ankle, Lower Leg	119	297	298
Therapeutic Exercise – Knee and Thigh	120	299	300
Therapeutic Exercise – Hip	121	301	302
Therapeutic Exercise – Back and Neck	122	303	304

Index

Athletic Training Clinical Education Guide is an activity and reference book designed to maximize student learning during clinical education. The Guide is written for all levels of athletic training students, beginner to advanced, who are gaining experience at a variety of clinical education settings such as schools, clinics, or physician's offices and working with an array of patients: high school athlete, active adult, professional athlete, and others. Because of the variety of activities and the completeness of the content, students are encouraged to use the book not with a single course but rather as a companion to their entire clinical education experience. Because of its assistance to Clinical Instructors, CIs are encouraged to keep a copy with them so they can make all clinical experiences learning experiences.

Concept

The real-life, chaotic structure of clinical education provides wonderful learning opportunities. However, the student and clinical instructor need to know how to recognize the real-life experiences as learning experiences. I wrote this book to provide a framework for learning in clinical education. We have an excellent framework for didactic education. This is an attempt to provide one for clinical education. It is my hope that this book will assist both students and instructors in improving student learning. Throughout my career as an athletic training educator I have continuously searched for ways to make clinical experiences learning experiences. This book is a compilation of those efforts.

Organization

The Guide is organized into four sections. Section 1 *Using this Book* provides the background information needed to take full advantage of the learning activities in the book. Chapter 2 *What is Reflection?* provides an in-depth explanation of how to reflect. I recommend that students read this chapter a couple of times so they thoroughly understand how to reflect. Students who learn to reflect well will find this to be one of the most valuable lifelong learning skills they can possess. Section 2 *Athletic Training Educational Competencies* is organized to include the content of the *Athletic Training Educational Competencies* 4th Ed. This section provides many activities that ensure clinical experiences become learning experiences. It also provides charts to record learning over time. Each chapter follows the same format:

Background Knowledge – In order for students to benefit from a clinical experience they must have the requisite knowledge. For this reason the accrediting agency (CAATE) requires didactic education prior to clinical experience. This section serves as a reminder to the student and the instructor of the knowledge a student needs in order to maximize his/her learning experience.

Goals – An active learner gets more out of an educational experience than a passive learner. Writing goals ensures that the student is actively engaged in the learning experience. Goals also serve as a check for the clinical instructor. Goals should match the experience. A mismatch between student written goals and potential clinical experiences allows the instructor to adjust the student expectation for the experience.

Discussion between Student and Clinical Instructor – Clinical instructors have valuable experience to share with their students. These experiences do not always reveal themselves as injury management situations. There is a great deal the clinical instructor can share with the student about policy, practice, and concerns. There may also be a great deal to share about events that happened in the clinical instructor's life prior to the student being placed with that instructor. This section provides the prompts that can be used to facilitate discussion and learning.

Reflection – In order to maximize learning from practical experiences students must use a process that allows them to recognize and internalize new information. Reflection helps transition physical experiences into learning experiences. Without reflection people live but do not learn. Reflection is such an important tool that Chapter 2 *Reflection* is devoted solely to teaching students how to reflect. Chapter 3 *Sample Reflection Assignments and Assessment Rubrics* is written for the benefit of both students and instructors. The better informed the student is about the learning and assessment process, the more likely he/she will be an active learner. The better the instructor understands the reflection process, the better he/she will be able to prompt and guide reflections.

Skills – For skills to become part of their repertoire athletic trainers need to practice their profession. Skills are organized into charts that allow verification of Learning Over Time. Each chart is designed to show progression from those skills demonstrated in isolation to multiple skills that are integrated into real-life athletic training practice.

Challenge Assignments – Athletic trainers integrate a great deal of knowledge and skill as they perform their jobs. Sometimes they need great people skills to accomplish a task. Sometimes their organizational skills are taxed as they manage large amounts of information. The Challenge Assignments provide an opportunity to insert real problems/tasks that athletic trainers manage. Having students complete these assignments gives them a realistic understanding of how all their knowledge and skill can be integrated into a single activity.

Journal – Writing down their thoughts helps students to solidify their thinking. Journaling is a more a free form of writing than the previously described reflection. There is no template to follow or question to answer. Journaling is simply students talking about and reacting to their own experiences. Journaling is part of this book for two reasons. First, athletic trainers communicate through writing quite often. Practice helps this process become efficient and effective. Second, journaling provides an opportunity for students to learn lessons that are important but were not necessarily planned. For example, in writing about injury management they may discover that the real challenge was dealing with people.

Section 3 *Reference Material* provides quick reference information for athletic training students. These chapters provide ample quiz material as students prepare for the BOC examination. Since clinical experience is not always filled with action, students can use this material to quiz each other. Section 4 *Rubrics* provides skill assessment rubrics. The rubrics are developed around the skills of athletic training but are differentiated for novice and advanced athletic training students. Because educators expect students to improve their knowledge and skill, they have different standards for novice and advanced students. These rubrics allow educators to assess the student at the appropriate level.

Features and Benefits

The Guide is unique because it organizes clinical experiences into learning experiences like no other text. Specifically it:

1. Can be used by novice and advanced students in all clinical rotations.
2. Incorporates all the Athletic Training Educational Competencies so the program can document Learning Over Time.
3. Is thorough enough to include all entry-level athletic training skills yet flexible enough to allow each program and instructor to emphasize what is important to them.
4. Teaches students how to direct their own learning through the use of Goals, Reflections, and Discussion questions.
5. Provides grading rubrics to help instructors and students assess clinical skills for both the novice and advanced student.
6. Provides students with in-depth, real-life challenge assignments to improve their critical thinking.
7. Includes reference material to assist student preparation for the BOC examination.

Online Instructor's Companion

Instructors will find an online companion, which includes quizzes and scenarios. The quizzes are intended to be used at the beginning of each chapter in Section 2 to help instructors decide if students have requisite knowledge for that content. The scenarios are written to provide help to instructors who are assessing athletic training skills. The middle column of the Learning Over Time chart is intended to be used with simulations. The scenarios should provide a starting point for instructors. Finally, the online companion provides a matrix that allows programs to compile all student skills. This is a convenient way to have a permanent record of skills and also a way to demonstrate learning over time for accreditation purposes. For convenience I suggest that instructors use the physical book to record student skill accomplishment. During breaks (Christmas, between rotations, etc.) the books can be turned into the Program Director for each student's skill assessment to be entered onto the matrix.

The online companion can be accessed at www.delmar.cengage.com/companions.

Feedback

There is an email link on the *Athletic Training Clinical Education Guide* online companion. I invite your comments and feedback on any aspect of the book or Web site. My goal is to make adjustments so this Guide will provide the structure needed to make clinical experiences learning experiences for all students.

I hope students and clinical instructors find this Guide helpful in providing some structure to the chaotic environment of clinical education. Practical experience has potential to be a very rich learning opportunity for students. As long as students and instructors continuously look for learning opportunities, they will find them.

Tim

ACKNOWLEDGMENTS

No significant project is completed in isolation. This book is no exception. All my professors, mentors, peers, and students have influenced me. Thank you. Your influence has been recorded in some way in these pages.

A special thank-you goes to my current and former students. This project got started because I wanted a way to make your clinical experience a deep learning experience. As you worked through assignments and asked me questions, you helped me make adjustments for the next group of students. The continuous feedback and scenarios you experienced solidified this project along the way. Thus your experience and feedback helped teach students who came after you. Your questions also helped me learn. Thank you for helping me learn and grow as an athletic trainer. I hope you got as much out of our interaction as I did.

My family, Susan, Jacob, Sarah, Chase, and Quinn, also deserves a thank-you. Because I want to be a good husband and father, I practice reflection as I describe in this book. Every decision I make that involves you causes me to ask myself if that was the right one. I know that I need to continue to grow in my role in our family just as I need to continue to grow as a professional. Like my students, you have provided me with constant experiences upon which to evaluate myself. Thanks for just being you. That has been enough to force me to reflect and grow – I hope.

Thanks to Delmar for making this project a reality. Matt Seeley saw potential in this book when others did not quite understand where this book would fit in. Thanks for your foresight and encouragement. Darcy Scelsi provided the guidance and feedback to help transform my thoughts and ideas into an organized work that communicated to the reader. Thanks.

Barbara Blackstone, BS, MSS
University of Maine, Presque Isle
Presque Isle, Maine

Hugh W. Harling, EdD, LAT, ATC
Methodist University
Fayetteville, North Carolina

Timothy G. Howell, EdD, ATC, CSCS
Alfred University
Alfred, New York

Jan Kiilsgaard, MS, ATC, LAT
Southern Arkansas University
Magnolia, Arkansas

Mark Lafferty, PhD, Med
Delaware Technical and Community College
Dover, Delaware

Karen M. Lew, Med, ATC, LAT
Southeastern Louisiana University
Hammond, Louisiana

William T. Lyons, MS, ATC
University of Wyoming
Laramie, Wyoming

Brendon R. McDermott, MS, ATC
University of Connecticut
Storrs, Connecticut

Carrie Meyer, PhD
Fort Lewis College
Durango, Colorado

Robert Stow, PhD, ATC, CSCS
University of Wisconsin – Eau Claire
Eau Claire, Wisconsin

Adam J. Thompson, PhD, ATC, LAT
Indiana Wesleyan University
Marion, Indiana

Sean Willeford, MS, ATC, LAT
Texas Christian University
Forth Worth, Texas

Dr. Laurent currently serves as Associate Dean for Academic Affairs at Lynchburg College in Virginia. Prior to this position he served as Department Chair for Athletic Training and Exercise Physiology at the same institution. Tim received his Bachelor of Science in Athletic Training from Indiana University; his Master of Science in Athletic Training from the University of Arizona; and his Doctor of Education in Education Administration from Ball State University. Between his master's and doctorate he served as Head Athletic Trainer at Saint Mary's University in Winona, Minnesota, and Head Athletic Trainer and Instructor at the University of Wisconsin – LaCrosse. In his twenty years as an athletic trainer he has continuously tried to make clinical education a valuable learning experience for his students. This book is a culmination of many clinical education teaching strategies he has used over the years.

At first glance it may appear that Associate Dean is very different from Athletic Trainer. In reality they are not that different. An athletic trainer communicates with many different people: coaches, parents, physicians, athletes, other athletic trainers, and others. This communication requires an understanding of the needs of the audience both from what information they need and the language/style they need for comprehension of the information. The Associate Dean works with a variety of audiences also: parents, students, faculty, administrators, trustees, and others. This also requires an understanding of the audience and their need for information. Both are helping positions. Both positions require patience when working with constituents who may be emotional or see the world from a different perspective than the Athletic Trainer or Administrator. Athletic training with all its requirements was a great preparatory experience for administration.

Using This Book

CHAPTER 1

How to Use This Book

Teach a student about Athletic Training and you prepare her for the next test.

Teach her how to learn from her experiences and you have taught her to be a lifelong learner.

The Structure of Athletic Training Programs

Athletic training, like other health care professions, uses a bipartite curriculum (a combination of classroom learning and hands-on learning). The reason for including both didactic (classroom learning) and clinical (hands-on) experience in entry-level education is to ensure that students possess both the knowledge and skill to function as competent professionals. Didactic education is designed to provide the science and reasoning behind athletic training knowledge. Clinical education is designed to provide the opportunity to apply athletic training knowledge and skill. The combination of these two education formats should provide an excellent learning opportunity for students to fully comprehend entry-level athletic training knowledge and skills. This dual approach should also provide a realistic view of the profession and help instill confidence in young professionals.

The Didactic Approach

Didactic education provides a formal structure in which information is presented, reviewed, applied, and assessed. Didactic education is considered an efficient way of delivering and evaluating knowledge because one instructor can teach many students simultaneously. This structured format allows for conversation among many students and the teacher. Classroom education also allows feedback for students and the teacher to indicate the level of learning that has occurred. Because a class can be repeated and content standardized, comparisons can be made between current and prior students. The formalized structure of didactic education allows monitoring of input (content and delivery) and output (knowledge and skill); thus effectiveness can be determined. Within athletic training, didactic education is the best way to show inclusion of educational competencies. However, formalization, structure, and efficiency come at the expense of "reality." Athletic Trainers make decisions about the severity of an injury and the course of treatment during a practice or game when others are watching and questioning what they do. Real situations are filled with uncertainty and lack the sterility that accompanies didactic education.

The Clinical Approach

Clinical education attempts to prepare a student for "the real world" by using not the classroom but the "lab" as the learning environment. The lab may be an actual room with athletic training (AT) equipment, but it may also be any practical setting. Examples of AT labs include the AT facilities, the tennis court, football field, or operating room. These labs provide the opportunity to integrate knowledge and skills into real life or simulated scenarios. Clinical education starts from the premise that learning in action is a good learning experience. With relatively little structure students must build their own structure around learning opportunities that present themselves. In the real world of athletic training, injury management is integrated with athletic training policy; prevention strategies and communication skills rely on each other; and job satisfaction and budget may be intertwined. Clinical education provides an opportunity for students to see that AT knowledge is not practiced in the compartments in which didactic education is delivered. This educationally chaotic environment may be overwhelming and confusing for many, but with proper guidance, clinical education helps students learn how to integrate their entire repertoire of AT knowledge and skill into the practice of AT.

Using This Book

Practical experience is a wonderful teaching tool; however, we need some assistance in ensuring that our practical experiences are learning experiences. This book includes learning activities and reference material. It is intended to accompany the student to clinical assignments. Activities and assignments are designed to help students involve as many senses as possible in learning clinical information. The more senses involved in the learning process, the deeper

the learning experience. When time allows, students should review reference material or converse with Clinical Instructors (CIs) about their athletic training experiences. Prior to a clinical rotation students should develop goals and perform a self-assessment. Throughout the rotation the student should reflect, practice skills, and complete complementary assignments. If students develop the ability to learn in the chaotic, clinical environment, they will be able to learn on their own.

Section 1 – Using This Book

Section 1 contains Chapters 1, 2, and 3. These chapters help the student and faculty understand how to use this book to facilitate learning.

Section 2 – Athletic Training Educational Competencies

Chapters in this section are divided into the content areas presented in the 4th Edition of the *Athletic Training Educational Competencies*. Within each chapter students are presented with several activities to assist them in learning AT content. Each chapter contains background knowledge, goals, discussion between student and instructor, reflection, skills verification, challenge assignments, and journaling. The chapters are placed in the order in which the content is presented in *Athletic Training Educational Competencies,* 4th Ed. This is likely not the order of any particular curriculum or any student's experience. Expect to jump around in completing the chapters in Section 2.

Background Knowledge

If you don't know what you don't know, you have no way of knowing what you need to know.

This section informs students of what they should know in order to get the most out of the learning experiences in this chapter. Clinical experiences are designed for students to utilize their knowledge and skill. Without foundation knowledge students will not be able to maximize their learning opportunities. Background Knowledge helps to prime students' thinking and motivate them to learn/relearn information they cannot quickly recall. With a solid foundation of background knowledge students will be able to utilize their knowledge to move closer to entry-level competence.

✔ Student Tips

Give yourself a quiz. How would you rate your knowledge/skill in this area? Are you ready for this content? If not, what are you going to do?

THE OBJECTIVES OF THIS BOOK ARE THE FOLLOWING:

1. Provide a framework for learning during clinical experiences.
2. Provide a checklist for Athletic Training skills.
3. Provide reference material for quick access during clinical experiences.
4. Provide discussion, reflection, and homework activities to facilitate learning during clinical experience.
5. Ensure learning over time and provide evidence of learning over time.
6. Evaluate student progress.
7. Integrate the 4th Edition of *Athletic Training Educational Competencies,* into clinical education.
8. Provide a framework for clinical skill assessment while allowing program flexibility to clinical instructors and students.
9. Teach students how to be lifelong learners.

✔ Instructor Tips

Use this section to guide assignments and discussion. Give an introductory quiz to determine students' level of background knowledge. If background knowledge is not at the appropriate level, use many of the chapter activities. If student knowledge is appropriate, assess skills and help students progress to the challenge activities. Instructors can refer to the online instructor guide for sample quizzes.

Goals

Goals provide direction. Educational goals provide direction to our education.

Writing goals forces self-evaluation. A good goal is one written with thorough analysis of what a person knows and can do in relation to what he needs to know or be able to do. By writing goals, students help construct a frame to learn from their clinical experiences. Goals direct and guide students to help them take ownership of their learning. Ownership increases meaning and ultimately advances professional development. As students consider their goals they should review them with their ACI/CI to be sure that they are realistic for the clinical experience and specific enough to be assessed.

An example of a poor and a good goal might help. Kara is a sophomore starting her first AT rotation. She has no experience with football. She thinks she needs to learn more about football in order to be a good ATC. This rotation is her opportunity. She crafts a goal which states: *I want to know more about football*. This goal is well intentioned but poorly written. It provides very little direction. A better goal might be written as: *By the end of this rotation I want to be able to describe to my roommate the typical injuries that occur to football players in each position*. This goal is better because not only is she specific about what she wants to learn, but she has also assigned the task of communicating that information to her roommate.

Kara might not be able to articulate the better goal. Without experience she may not know that the different football positions have different physical demands and thus different typical injuries. But if she at least starts with the first goal and then discusses her goal with the clinical instructor, the instructor can help her match her needs with the clinical experience.

✔ Student Tips

If you are having trouble writing goals, review the Background Knowledge and the Skills assigned to the chapter. Filling in the holes in your knowledge and ability can lead you to a worthwhile goal.

✔ Instructor Tips

Help students form goals by considering their typical problems. Also consider the struggles you had as you were learning the content in each area. Be sure the students' goals match the experience you have to offer.

Discussion between the Student and ACI/CI

Smart people learn from books and teachers. Wise people learn from their experiences and the experiences of others.

The clinical instructor has a lifetime of experience. Students should learn from the experiences of their ACI/CIs. This section provides conversation material for the ACI/CI and student. It also helps to provide some structure to the conversation so that specific content from each chapter is covered. Discussion allows for deep review of experiences that may have happened long ago or may have spanned a period that would normally extend beyond a clinical rotation. Discussion is very important to student learning because it allows the students to develop and articulate thoughts and ideas about situations which they have not yet experienced.

✔ Student Tips

Develop questions based on what you know and do not know in conjunction with the clinical experience. This is your opportunity to pick the brain of your instructor. Try to know all of your instructor's experiences.

✔ Instructor Tips

Think of other questions in each area. Remember the struggles you had as a student. Pose questions that you wish you had asked as a student.

Reflection

Those who do not reflect upon their experiences are sentenced to repeat failures and are prevented from repeating successes.

Reflection is performed after a student experiences athletic training. The reflection questions ask the student to think about what happened and analyze the situation. Reflection ensures that the experience is not the learning finale but rather the stimulus for further learning and future development. Questions in this section cover a broad spectrum of experiences so students may not be able to answer all of them. The intention is not to have a perfect list of reflection questions but rather a list that is inclusive enough to cover many areas and teach students how to develop their own reflection questions. Chapter 2 contains a complete explanation of how to reflect.

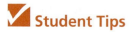

Student Tips

Each night make brief notes about your clinical experience. Attempt to record what you learned in addition to what you did.

Instructor Tips

Assign weekly reflection questions. The assignment can be emailed back to you. A specific reflection question can be assigned or students can choose the reflection that matches their experience. Ultimately you want students to develop their own reflections based on their clinical experience.

Skills – Learning Over Time Verification

Integrating knowledge and skill in the context of patient care makes an athletic trainer a professional.

The skills section provides an opportunity for students to demonstrate their athletic training skills. This section also provides a means of assessing skills. Some structure is provided to help direct the student; however, great freedom is provided to the ACI/CI in determining the specific skill to be performed. The ACI/CI also uses his/her professional judgment in determining the quality of the skill.

The first column "Skill" is a listing of athletic training skills students need to master. Note that there are extra blanks in this column. This is to allow the clinical instructor or student to add skills or more specifically delineate skills. The second column "Individual Skill" is designed to help ensure that the skill can be performed as an isolated skill. This is intended to help the student focus on the skill itself without the distraction of a real AT situation. The third column "Simulation/Random" allows larger chunks of information to be packaged together. For example, the clinical instructor might ask the student to demonstrate assessment of ankle range of motion. The student would need to determine which ranges need to be assessed and how to perform the skill. This column allows for spot checking and scenarios.

Scenarios allow the clinical instructor to determine the student's ability to integrate AT knowledge and skill without having a live patient. (Instructors can refer to the online guide for sample scenarios.) The final column "Integrated into AT" allows the student to integrate knowledge and skill into a real AT situation. An athletic training student may evaluate an injured patient. In her evaluation the student may emphasize

or deemphasize a portion of the evaluation based on feedback from the patient. Following a real situation in which the AT student acted, the clinical instructor should discuss the experience with the student. Questions to foster student self-analysis should be used. *Why did you ____? Why didn't you _____ ?* Integrating knowledge and skill into the practice of AT is the highest cognition level and should be encouraged.

This four-column system helps ensure higher level utilization of knowledge and skill. It also provides a means of demonstrating learning over time. Below the final line of the chart is a line for verification. The program can decide the level of verification needed. It can be self, peer, CI, ACI or other. The space below the charts is intentionally left blank. This space serves as a note page for students and instructors.

This chart helps to show **Learning Over Time** in two ways. First, the verification shows repeated exposures to the material. Second, with each exposure the task gets less mechanical and more real. The ideal situation is that the last column would be verified with a real patient suffering from an actual pathology. Please note that learning over time means there is a gap between the demonstrations of skills. The first signature may occur during the sophomore year, and the third signature may occur during the senior year. Programs may choose to use this as their assessment tool for the skills. Others may want to use the chart as practice and repeated exposure only (i.e., Learning Over Time) and use the rubrics in Section 4 as the assessment of the skill.

Student Tips

Practice the skills repeatedly. A good athletic trainer is a very skilled technician.

Instructor Tips

Describing how to perform a skill is a lower level of thinking than the student will ultimately need but is the appropriate starting point. As the student progresses be sure to ask "Why" questions. See the online instructor's guide for sample scenarios.

Challenge Assignments

In-depth exploration allows for in-depth learning.

While clinical experiences provide the primary learning stimulus in clinical education, there is great value in learning assignments that connect clinical experiences with reference material. These assignments are designed for the advanced student who is ready to assume more AT responsibility. Assignments require

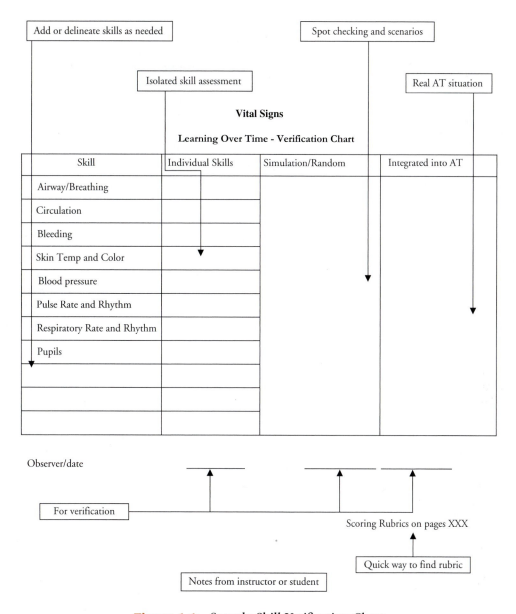

Figure 1.1 Sample Skill Verification Chart

students to collect, analyze, and synthesize information that can be used in clinical practice. Some assignments will be more germane than others to the students' experiences. However, all assignments are pertinent to the professional development of Athletic Trainers.

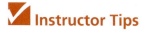 **Student Tips**

Tackle these assignments as though they were part of your employment. They may be part of your real work very soon.

Instructor Tips

Add assignments that are pertinent. Any of the projects you are involved with will be good learning projects for the students.

Journaling

Writing often solidifies learning.

Journaling helps experiences become learning experiences. The act of writing facilitates recall, which is the first step in learning from what we experience. Students can journal about anything. They will often learn about one topic (e.g., communication) when journaling about another topic (e.g., therapeutic exercise). Students are encouraged to use additional paper as needed and share their journal entries with other students and clinical instructors. However, journaling can be a very private endeavor. Students should know in advance if they will be expected to share their entries.

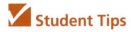
Student Tips

Take notes on what has helped you learn. Take advantage of this space to write notes to yourself.

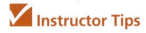
Instructor Tips

Point out unique, different, interesting experiences. Remember, students do not always know that an experience is unique. Helping by pointing out items which students can journal about will help them learn how to pay attention to learning opportunities.

Section 3 – Reference Material

Chapters in this section contain reference material. Students should take advantage of less busy clinical times to quiz each other on the content of these chapters. This section is intended to be a quick reference not a complete reference. Chapters should stand as reminders to the student and instructor of some of the information students should be able to recall quickly.

Section 4 – Rubrics

Scoring rubrics allow the instructor to assess the student on predetermined criteria. Rubrics make grading uniform and consistent. The rubrics for the novice AT student are designed for the person learning the skill. The most important assessment is on the mechanics of the skill. This approach is used because skills must be learned before results of skills can be interpreted. For example, a poorly performed Lachman's test provides no information about the integrity of the ACL. The skill must be solid before results can be meaningful.

The advanced student needs to transition to higher level thinking. Interpretation, modification, and explanation of skills are important to this person. A positive Lachman's test must be explained to the athlete and others. An initial positive test might need to be followed by a modified version of the test to verify results. Treatment options must be reviewed. The advanced AT student is a short step away from practicing athletic training. The advanced rubrics are designed to assess the student's ability to think as a practicing professional.

Student Tips

As a novice your responsibility is to learn all the steps of the skills and learn them properly. As an advanced student your responsibility is to combine skills in a way they would be displayed in a real situation. You need to progress your thinking, but you can only do this after you have a complete grasp of the skills in each area.

Instructor Tips

Expect novice students to demonstrate skills but do not attempt to distract them with too many questions. The advanced student should be able to operate effectively among multiple distractions. Use multiple rubrics together to create a realistic scenario. For example, if a patient has a femur fracture the athletic trainer needs to assess both the person's leg and vital signs. It is not possible to include rubrics to cover all possible situations, but because real situations require integration of multiple skills and knowledge sets instructors should combine rubrics.

Reflection

Those who do not reflect upon their experiences are sentenced to repeat failures and are prevented from repeating successes.

What is Reflection?

Athletic Trainers are very busy rushing from one practice, event, or evaluation to the next. In some situations ATs are so busy that they do not have time to think. Without looking back on what they have experienced, ATs can miss learning opportunities. When ATs fail to reflect on experiences they may not gain the knowledge to repeat successes or to avoid repeating failures.

Reflection is the process of recalling, analyzing, and synthesizing experiences in order to make them real; making note of strengths and weaknesses; and choosing behaviors to continue, discontinue, or modify. Reflection allows us to grow as professionals so that we do not have to be the same athletic trainer twenty years post-certification that we were twenty days post-certification. In short, reflection allows us to learn from our experiences. With reflection we gain knowledge from our experience. Without reflection we take up time in our life with activities but do not grow as we should. Adapting an idea from the Spanish philosopher George Santayana, those who do not study history are doomed to repeat it. Those who do not reflect on their own history are doomed to repeat mistakes and forget the details that produced successes. Reflection helps us prepare for, succeed in, and learn from our experiences. The required clinical

experience in athletic training provides the exposure to the profession needed by students to help them learn to integrate knowledge and skill into their professional repertoire.

Reflection is no different from any other skill. It takes practice in order to perform well. The reflection questions in each chapter provide an opportunity for students to learn from their experiences. The hope is that students will continue to use reflection as a learning tool so they can learn from their experiences throughout their entire athletic training career. Learning to reflect is similar to learning to tape an ankle. Initially, great effort is needed to recall the proper steps. Next, the student focuses on applying the tape without wrinkles. Finally, after taping enough ankles, the athletic training student can tape well without thinking about the task of taping. Now the athletic trainer can use his/her mental ability to dual task. It is not uncommon for an experienced athletic trainer to tape one athlete while taking the history of another injured athlete.

Initially, reflection will take conscious effort. The best way to ensure that students are consciously reflecting is for them to write down the reflection. This allows the student and instructor to assess the reflection. As a person becomes competent in reflection it will become natural. The reflective learner will be able to reflect during and after experiences to learn from them. In the end, all experiences will be learning or refining experiences.

Reflection is most powerful when it is directly linked to an event a person has experienced. For example, this book could be a list of scenarios encountered by athletic trainers. Students could be asked to evaluate the situation and state what they would do. But generic scenarios facilitate learning only to a point. Reflecting upon their own experiences makes a situation real, providing more meaning and learning opportunities.

How to Reflect

Like any new knowledge or skill, reflection needs to be taught and learned in order to be used. The first step in the learning process is for the information to be explained. Next, a demonstration of how to use the information helps the student put the knowledge or skill into context. Finally, the new skill must be practiced. This chapter explains the reflection process. It also provides sample reflections and assesses the examples presented. The practice is up to the student. The more the student understands the reflection process and the more he/she practices, the easier reflection will become and the greater the gains. Thorough reflection includes three steps:

Step 1: Recall – a list of What Happened.

Step 2: Analyze – an explanation of So What.

Step 3: Synthesize – a determination of Now What.

Including these three components into a reflection helps ensure that practical experiences are learning experiences.

Recall – What Happened?

The first and most important reflection step is recall. By acknowledging what happened, recall allows analysis and synthesis of experiences. During recall the student may:

• Replay the experience mentally or on paper.

• Recount the details of a conversation.

• Visualize how a technique or treatment was applied.

• Remember hand placement during a technique or treatment.

• List all the steps in an evaluation of an injured athlete.

Recall makes students pay attention to what they experienced and learned. Sometimes a list is all that is needed to help people learn from their experience.

How to Recall

Take about 10 – 15 minutes at the conclusion of the day to recall your experiences. You may wish to write

them down or you may wish to make notes in outline or phrase format. You can take mental notes, but it is better to solidify your thoughts on paper until recall becomes routine. Recall even the events that do not seem remarkable. They may be very important later. Every ATC can tell you of several minor events that resulted in big consequences. The consequences may have been big because the injury was actually more severe than it initially appeared or because the reaction of the coach, athlete, parent, community, etc. required great effort from the ATC. For example, nonspecific bone pain could end up being a very serious pathology such as cancer. The diagnosis of cancer may come a long time after the initial complaint of vague pain in the leg. You will want to learn as much as possible about all situations, so that the next time you encounter a similar situation you will have appropriate knowledge to deal with the pathology or problem. Recall helps you learn because it stimulates your interest and makes you cognizant of the things you need to learn. When you recall ask yourself:

• What happened?

• When did it happen?

• What was happening around me?

Asking these questions helps you recall all events. Some events will be significant. Others may not be so important. One challenge is to recall all events and not just those that appear to be germane to the main situation. Typically a person will not automatically recognize every important event as important at the time it happens. This is why thorough recall is necessary. Later analysis and synthesis can determine the significance of the information.

A second challenge is being objective when recalling events. Objective recall allows replaying events from multiple perspectives. Objectivity is critical in confrontational situations. Without being objective you will only see things from your perspective, limiting your ability to learn how others think. Lack of objectivity also prevents critical analysis of your own actions. To determine if you are objective, answer these questions:

• Would others recall the events the same way?

• If I was sharing my recall of the events of yesterday, would others agree?

• When I recall what I said, does it now sound offensive?

Be honest when you answer these questions. If you want to grow as a professional, you must be able to be objective and learn from both positive and negative experiences. Most situations are not confrontational, but those that are pose a challenge to objectivity.

One way to learn to be objective is to recall another person's actions. Since observation students are observing and not practicing athletic training skills, they are in a very good position to use recall to learn about athletic training. Recall helps students determine what athletic trainers do and how people react to their actions. With practice, students will be ready to more appropriately evaluate their own actions and decisions.

Practice

This exercise will help you improve your recall skills. Think of one athletic training situation you encountered yesterday. If the situation was an injured patient, recall the complaint, the reaction of the patient, the questions from the clinical instructor, the response of the patient to the questions, and the physical examination performed. These are the things to which people usually pay attention. Now recall the body language used by the patient and the clinician. Did the patient answer in long or short responses? Did the patient have any scars or atrophy distal to the injury? What time was it? Was a coach, parent, or friend present? What were they doing? Were there any extraneous conditions that affected this particular situation? When you are efficient at recalling, you can take mental notes of all happenings without interfering with your concentration on the task at hand.

Sample

Below is a sample reflection. As you read this reflection, identify the information recalled. Is the recall thorough enough for you to learn something?

> I started my rotation at the doctor's office this week. It's been a very positive experience so far. I learned one thing that was important. When a patient complains of discomfort, we need to look at the broad spectrum instead of just focusing on the complaint. At the doctor's office, a patient complained of pain in his foot with numbness from time to time. The occupation of the patient involved standing still for many hours, and he has rigid feet. An X-ray was taken to rule out bone spurs. Since diabetes can cause numbness in the extremities, blood sugar was assessed. The patient also had negative dermatome and myotome tests. This information is useful in the sense that it can detect many illnesses. If an athlete comes into the athletic training room and complains of numbness and pain in the extremities and all the dermatomes and myotomes are negative, we might send the athlete to the health center for a blood sugar test just to rule out other illness. A certain complaint can be indicative of some other illness. We need to do the tests to rule out other possibilities.

Notice how several pieces of information were reported. He recalled the patient's complaint of foot pain and numbness, the occupational requirements of the patient, the use of diagnostic X-ray, the physician's concern about diabetes, the administration of a blood sugar level test, and negative results of dermatome and myotome assessment. This amount of recall is very good. Because so much information was recalled, he was able to indicate the significance of this experience. He learned to be cognizant of pathologies that may contribute to foot pain. Thorough recall of information sets the stage for learning from this experience.

Analyze – So What?

Analyzing an event requires evaluating your actions and the actions of others in the context of the situation. Doing so allows you to determine So What. This helps put things into perspective so you realize how one situation is similar to or different from other situations. For example, injury evaluations performed by various people may look different. An injury assessment performed by a sophomore athletic training student may include an acceptable history of the injury. The student may ask all the standard history questions, and these questions will likely reveal some pertinent information. In following the format learned in class the history questions are likely somewhat generic and disconnected from each other. But an experienced ATC may understand the daily routine of the cross country team and ask a series of connected questions that paints a complete picture of the athlete's injury history. He may have a better understanding of how the daily workouts typically affect freshmen runners. As a result of experience and knowledge, the ATC's questions may be very specific to the runner's conditioning program. The ATC will likely dig deeper into the athlete's responses and allow one question to lead to another as he gets clarification from the athlete. As you analyze these two evaluations, you should notice specifically *how* one evaluation is more advanced than the other, not simply that it *is* more advanced.

How to Analyze

Effective analysis provides meaning to your experiences. Analysis should show some evidence of understanding. It should also show evidence of self-awareness or awareness of others. Look at your list of events that you recalled from a clinical experience. Determine if the events were normal, abnormal, right, wrong, good, bad, etc. compared to what you know and expect. Analyze your actions and the actions of others. Ask yourself:

• Did I miss anything?

• Could I have done better?

• Did my actions, words, or body language elicit the response I wanted?

• What would an experienced ATC have done?

Compare and contrast experiences to what you have read and what you have been told. The more you know, the more thorough your analysis can be and the more critical you should be. That means a freshman has relatively little knowledge and experience upon which to analyze her actions. A senior, however, should be able to analyze her experiences from multiple perspectives with insight into many experiences. The more experience a person has, the more she realizes that her analysis leads to more questions. The world simultaneously becomes clearer and more ambiguous. Although you may not be an experienced ATC, you should aspire to emulate those who represent the profession well. Analysis is critical to determining how you should adjust your actions so you can be the ATC you want to be.

One challenge to effective analysis is to avoid the habit of using dichotomous terms in your final analysis. Analyzing as "good" or "bad" does not help you to use the information. These dichotomous terms do not help you know what to do and what not to do. Analysis should help you understand why people (including you) behave as they do. For example, a very knowledgeable Head ATC was not viewed favorably by his students and patients. His assessment and prescriptions would rival those of the best ATCs and physicians in the country. The problem was that he communicated with everyone the same way. His brief, accurate, anatomical explanations were just right for busy physicians and ATCs. These same explanations to athletes and students were not well received. Athletes and students were often left with their mouths hanging open, wondering what he said. Students got in the habit of asking another ATC to interpret what the Head ATC said. When students had questions, they avoided the Head ATC. A superficial analysis reveals bad communication with athletes and students. A thorough analysis reveals why and how there was a communication gap between the Head ATC and others. The real problem was that the Head ATC communicated with everyone the same way, even though some people did not have the background knowledge to understand him. Athletes and students labeled the Head ATC as a poor athletic trainer. From their perspective, a good athletic trainer would be able to explain things using terms they could understand.

A second challenge is to analyze a situation from multiple perspectives. What comments would a patient make about a particular situation? How would the coach, parent, teammates, administrators, peers, and the public evaluate the situation? It is important that you can evaluate situations from multiple perspectives because you will be judged throughout your career. Sometimes the judging will be a formal arrangement to determine your job performance. At other times the judging will be from someone who wants to pass on his opinion to your administrator. You need to know that judgments are always from the perspective of the judge, so it is to your advantage to understand how people think. As people judge you they may conclude that you are effective, ineffective, or indifferent as an athletic trainer. They may use criteria that are germane to your ability to function as an athletic trainer like knowledge and skill. They may use professional behaviors such as communication skills and conduct. Or they may use criteria that are important to them but unimportant to you. For example, a coach may determine that you are a competent athletic trainer because you keep athletes on the field. A peer may have the opposite opinion because you rush people back to the field too soon.

Another challenge to effective analysis is being accurate and thorough. Saying you are good or bad at something is not sufficient. You must specify how you compare to others. An ATC may know that he does not communicate well with coaches. He may know this because he does not have a good relationship with a particular coach. If he really wants to progress to the next step of synthesizing (i.e., using this information), he must compare his actions to what other ATCs do when they work with difficult people. The ATC may like to communicate via email because it is efficient. He can send email messages from home at night or in the morning. This system may be efficient because he does not have to find the coach or take time out of his day. However, this means of communicating may not work well if the coach prefers to communicate face to face. An honest analysis reveals that this ATC's chosen means of communicating is not the best means of communicating with this particular coach.

Practice

Write an analysis of one of your clinical experiences. Have someone read it and mark which of the criteria for analysis your reflection satisfies. Your reflection can satisfy many criteria.

_____ Makes a comparison

_____ Puts a situation into context

_____ Helps others understand your thinking

_____ Explains why you did or did not do something

_____ Explains what you learned

_____ Explains why something is right, wrong, typical, atypical, etc.

_____ Explains a situation from a perspective other than yours as a student

If your analysis does not meet one or more of these criteria, you probably did not analyze the situation. One common problem students have is putting additional words into their recall rather than providing meaning to their reflection.

Sample

Below is a sample reflection. As you read, assess the analysis using the criteria from the practice analysis above to determine the quality of his analysis.

How has your perception of athletic training changed during your time as an athletic training student (ATS)?

> When I came in as an ATS I never really realized just what the profession of athletic training required. My first perceptions of the profession were the outer layers. I viewed athletic training as a profession of caring for athletes. But now I realize just how deep the profession goes. Not only do athletic trainers have responsibilities to the athletes but they also have them to the profession, coaches, parents, and other medical professions. Athletic training is a much more time consuming profession than I realized. Not only are the working hours irregular, but often times athletic trainers are required to put far more time into administration matters on top of caring for athletes and covering practices and games. All this being said, my outlook on the profession still has not changed. Even though the hours are usually long and irregular and the pay is not exceptional, I still see the profession as the right one for me.

Notice how this student explained the demands of athletic training. He compared his initial perception (superficial) to his later perception (deep). His initial perception was that athletic trainers cared for athletes. Now he realizes that athletic trainers have responsibilities to many other people and tasks. The student concludes that athletic training is still right for him. He made a before and after comparison. He helped others understand his thoughts on the profession by explaining what he learned about the responsibilities of ATCs. This is a very good analysis because it shows an in-depth understanding of athletic training. It also emphasizes the need for students to experience athletic training for themselves. This student most likely heard ATCs talk about irregular hours, administrative tasks and low pay before, but that talk from his teachers did not mean as much as his own experience with athletic training. His experience gave meaning to what he had heard before.

Synthesize – Now What?

Synthesis is the process of pulling things together so we can use information. It is answering the question, Now what? A teacher synthesizes information when she teaches a class. She combines research, text information, personal experience, peer experience and other sources of information to develop a presentation for the class. A class period may take the form of a PowerPoint presentation, class discussion, case studies, or any other approach that she deems appropriate. In designing the class, the teacher has synthesized the information into a useable form for the students. In this case, synthesis has resulted in creating a class. Students synthesize information to create papers, give presentations, or complete projects. Our clinical experience provides us with the opportunity to integrate athletic training knowledge with athletic training skills so we can develop into competent professionals. Without synthesizing our experiences, we are not maximizing our learning opportunities.

Synthesis can also help us confirm our actions. We do not always have to create new information. Sometimes we are doing the right things. Through the processes of recall, analysis, and synthesis, we may conclude that our actions are the best actions for us. An example of this to which most students can relate is ankle taping. At first you learned what to include in the ankle taping procedure because you recalled the appropriate steps. Next you analyzed your taping. You may have concluded that you had more wrinkles than some classmates and fewer wrinkles than others. You continued to practice and get feedback from others until you learned how to apply a heel lock at the proper angle to avoid wrinkles. You then made adjustments so that you could apply the tape at the correct angle on any foot—right, left, large, small, bony, fleshy, etc. You synthesized your experiences to create a tape job that was consistently neat and effective. Now that you have this skill, you synthesize your experiences to confirm that you still apply the tape properly.

Synthesis is the hardest part of reflection because in combining information you are putting things together in a distinct way, so they work for you. In this respect, synthesis is a personalized process. There is no one right way to practice athletic training. You need to find the way that works for you. You have to take the best from all you know, with the resources and limitations you have, to create your own distinct system. For example, after you have conducted mass physicals for the first, second, or third time you should revisit the process to determine if there is a way to make conducting physicals better. In your reflection you should consider specific problems and limitations you encountered.

How to Synthesize

Now that you have recalled information and analyzed it, how will you use the information? Ask yourself:

- If I was to repeat this scenario, what would I do the same or differently?

- How will I ensure that I repeat my successes and avoid repeating my failures?

- What would be the ideal reaction from all involved?

For example, imagine that you instructed a patient on performing step-up exercises as part of rehabilitation. In your instructions you showed him the proper way to complete the step up but did not emphasize knee position. This just did not enter your mind as a point to emphasize. Then, as you watch, you notice that the athlete is getting to the top of the step, but his leg is falling into a valgus position. You conclude that he was not engaging the external hip rotators as he stepped. This lack of synergistic contraction caused his knee to fall into a position that placed undue stress on the articulating surface of the patella. As part of your synthesis of this situation you make a mental note to 1) emphasize knee position during the step up and 2) to include hip external rotation strengthening in knee rehabilitation programs.

A challenge in synthesizing information is not to conclude that the process is over just because you synthesized information one time. We must continuously reevaluate what we do to determine what we should do next. If we make the assumption that what we did in the past was appropriate therefore our current actions are appropriate, we will miss an opportunity to better ourselves. Once we can synthesize (i.e., use information we recalled and analyzed) we can say we have "learned" something. As we get good at reflecting we will be able to progress through the reflection steps while we are working. We will not have to wait until later to reflect. Reflection in action allows us to make continuous adjustments so that we make the best decisions for each situation.

Practice

Below is a practice exercise. Take your time. Synthesis is the hardest step because it requires the most mental effort. Repeat this exercise with different clinical experiences until synthesis becomes a natural part of reflecting.

Write a reflection that shows evidence of synthesis. After you write your reflection, reread it to determine if you meet the following criteria. Then have someone else assess your reflection to determine if that person thinks you have synthesized your experience.

_____ Is there evidence of information being used?

_____ Is there evidence of confirmation of skills or knowledge?

_____ Is there evidence of how the information will be used in the future?

Sample

Below is an example of a reflection. As you read the reflection, attempt to determine how the student will behave in the future when she is presented with a difficult situation.

Why is problem solving an important skill for athletic trainers?

> While I was at baseball practice this week an athlete came up to us complaining of a wrist injury. His wrist would "pop" very loudly and obviously when he flexed or extended his wrist. We assumed that it was a ligament problem. We did other tests to try to figure out the problem, but it was very odd and Ann had never seen anything like it before. The athlete had had past medical history of laxity in his wrist but never this badly. As we sat there and looked at it, Ann started thinking that maybe it was his lunate. For example, when you sit back on your hands, when they are completely extended sometimes your wrist pops. Now she could be completely wrong here, but she thought maybe his lunate could be subluxing? Now neither she nor I knew if this was possible, but it made some sense to us. We have referred the athlete to a doctor. As I was thinking about my reflection question, I thought about how problem solving is so important in athletic training. Yes, we learn through books and other people, but in athletic training there is not always a textbook answer. Everything is different; one thing might work on one person, while not on another and something might be out of the ordinary for an individual when looking at an athlete just because that is how they are. Either way this experience reminded me sometimes that you have to bring all of your knowledge together and try to solve the problem or at least get a basis off of it. This skill cannot be taught to you. It can be helped in developing through practice and mentors, but experience is critical. Problem solving skills make athletic trainers stay on their toes and to be ready for pretty much anything or any situation.

This reflection is not only a good example of a student synthesizing information but also an excellent overview of the synthesis process. Notice how she realizes that problem solving is important. If you substitute "synthesis" for each time she says "problem solving" you will have a very good understanding of how the synthesis process works. We must continually synthesize our experiences. We need to create information based on pieces of information. This is what athletic trainers do. This is why synthesizing our clinical experiences is so important. This student has a personal example in her life to emphasize why synthesis is critical. I am confident she will never forget to synthesize information to solve problems.

Reflection – Putting It All Together

A well-written, thorough reflection should contain evidence of each of the reflection steps.

Recall – a list of What happened.

Analyze – an explanation of So What.

Synthesize – a determination of Now What.

It should be organized in such a way as to convey this information to the reader and most importantly to the student/author of the reflection. However, there is no requirement that the reflection be long or organized in the order of recall, analyze, and then synthesize. Any one of the reflection steps may be very short or drawn out depending on the number of words a student needs to Recall, Analyze, and Synthesize her thoughts. Students have different writing and thinking styles; therefore, students will have different reflection styles.

Sample

A final student reflection sample will illustrate how Recall, Analyze, and Synthesize can be put into a single reflection. Notice that although all three reflection components are included in this passage, Recall consumes the most words. Notice also that the student does not write in distinct sections but simply tells her story.

Today I was on the track with the field hockey team while they were running intervals. After running a sprint one of the girls asked me where Jane was. When I told her Jane was busy with another athlete she was annoyed. I asked her what was bothering her. She just said that it was her IT Band in a pissy sort of voice that kinda made me feel like I wasn't good enough to help her. I asked her if she wanted to be stretched and she agreed. When I was stretching her she wasn't able to get a stretch from any of the stretches, some were ones that had worked for her in the past and I tried a new one with her we had learned in class with no luck. She continued with practice. She came into the AT room after practice and wanted ultrasound which she hadn't had in over a week. I tried to explain to her that we didn't do ultrasound after practice, that it was considered a heat treatment and that it was only given before practice. She was still not happy and went immediately to the Head ATC who not only agreed with me, but also explained to the athlete that ultrasound was done on a regular basis, not just randomly. I think that the athlete left the AT room unhappy with both me and the Head ATC, but I also think that when she says something to Jane that Jane will tell her the same thing that I said.

This student recalled the events by listing What Happened. The athlete was a field hockey player. She was running intervals on the track. She had IT Band pain. Stretching did not work. And the athlete inquired about ultrasound. She then analyzed, So What, the use of US and stretching in this reflection: ". . .some were ones that had worked for her in the past and I tried a new one with her we had learned in class with no luck." She then confirmed her knowledge, Now What, when she asserted that the "head ATC… agreed with me" and "Jane will tell her the same thing that I said." She used all the elements of a thorough reflection, and she did it using her words and her writing (thinking) style.

The point of the reflection from this student was to confirm the student's knowledge of treating IT Band syndrome. She could have used the same situation to reflect upon communication; communication between the athlete and student, communication between the athlete and the Head ATC, or communication between the student and the Head ATC. Most of our clinical experiences teach or confirm our knowledge in many areas. The challenge is to learn as much as possible from every experience we have.

CHAPTER 3

Sample Reflection Assignments and Assessment Rubrics

Deep learning requires a thorough understanding of the learning process, not just the desired result.

Why This Is Important

This chapter presents reflection assignments and grading rubrics. The curious reader (I want you all to be curious) may be wondering why a chapter on sample assignments and assessment rubrics is included in this book. Isn't this information for teachers only? No, this information is not for teachers only. Students need to learn to think like teachers. They need to have a thorough understanding of the entire learning process. Deep understanding comes when learners can actively manipulate thoughts and ideas by "playing" with information. There should be no guessing by the students as to what a teacher is looking for in student work. But there is also another reason for the students to understand reflection from an assignment and grading perspective. After formal education is complete, learning is not finished. The better a professional knows the reflection process, the better learner he will be in this dynamic profession. In a couple of years today's student may be the clinical instructor. The cycle of learning from clinical experience is perpetuated when everyone understands reflection from the perspective of student and teacher.

Reflection Assignments

Reflection assignments can take multiple forms. Sample assignments illustrate how reflection can be used in the curriculum and provide a variety of practice opportunities. Reflection is not a single activity. It is a process that can be applied to many situations. Showing many ways in which to utilize this learning tool should help to stimulate thinking about how reflection can be applied to other learning experiences and in other environments. A student who can apply reflection to many facets of his life understands reflection much better than the student who can only use reflection in one way. A goal of this book is to get students to use reflection now as they learn about the profession of athletic training. A secondary goal of this book is to develop a lifelong learning habit that helps ATCs be competent, contributing professionals. Assignments provide practice. Practice helps refine our skills.

Rubrics

Rubrics allow students to assess their own reflection. This is no different from the checklists presented in

Chapter 2, *Reflection*. The checklists were based on indicators of recall, analysis, and synthesis, allowing students to assess the quality of their reflections. Thus students can reflect on their reflection. Grading rubrics provide students with tools to evaluate completed assignments. Remember, analysis is not only the second step in reflection. It is also the fourth, sixth, eighth, etc. We continuously analyze what we have synthesized so we can confirm our actions and determine necessary adjustments. Critiquing our own work is essential in helping us become self-learners.

Thinking Like an Instructor

Athletic training is a people profession. If we do not understand the people with whom we work, we will have a difficult time being successful and happy with our work. Students should understand how teachers think. Athletic trainers should understand how patients think. The premise is that athletic trainers can work with, deal with, and communicate better with people they understand. A student has a better chance for success if he can think like a teacher. Knowing *why* an assignment was given, *what* the teacher expects, and *how* the assignment will be assessed provides great insight that assists in successful completion of an assignment.

Reflection Assignments and Rubrics

Below are four sample assignments and accompanying rubrics. A discussion of the assignment and critique of the rubrics follow. These assignments are designed to accompany athletic training clinical experiences in all settings by all students. Modifications are encouraged to accommodate program objectives and student needs.

Sample Assignment #1 – Weekly Reflection

You will answer one reflection question per week. There is no particular order in which questions must be answered. Choose a reflection question that allows you to reflect upon your weekly experience. Questions can be answered more than once if a particular question has repeated relevance to your experiences as a student. You are also encouraged to pose and answer your own reflection questions. Posing and answering your own question indicates a thorough understanding of reflection. Be sure to include the question you are answering when you turn in your reflection. Email your reflections to the Program Director by Monday morning of each week. The total points earned will be included as part of your clinical education grade for the semester.

This assignment is ideal for beginning students because it helps accomplish two goals. It helps students get in the habit of reflecting on their clinical experiences, and it helps teach them how to reflect. It does this by having several mini-assignments. Mini-assignments allow for regular feedback without strong consequences for poor performance. If a student is having a difficult time reflecting at a level higher than recall, at least she will have plenty of feedback and opportunity to adjust her reflections. If a student completely forgets to complete an assignment (this happens to everyone) the overall grade will not be in jeopardy.

The best way to approach this assignment is to read all reflection questions first. Next, spend about 10 to 15 minutes each day recalling the events of the day. Take notes directly in the book after the appropriate question or chapter. On the weekend analyze the week's events. Synthesize your reflection into a single paragraph or two. Be sure to check each reflection to see if it meets the criteria for recall, analysis, and synthesis (see Chapter 2).

Although this assignment is quick and easy, reflections may take some time and effort at the beginning of the semester. Soon, however, students will learn the reflection process and apply it with little effort. Students will start to anticipate their reflection and will look for appropriate reflection opportunities. Before long the list of reflection questions in Chapters 4 through 16 will not be long enough. Students will begin writing their own questions.

Notice that the reflection is sent via email to the Program Director (PD). Bypassing the clinical instructor who works directly with the student and records the final grade is intentional. Occasionally students use reflections as a way to vent frustrations. This is an acceptable use of reflection as long as they have been thorough in their thoughts. Venting, however, can be at the expense of ATCs, ACIs, CIs, and others with whom students work. Students need to learn how to vent frustrations without being personal in their expressions. For this reason, reflection needs to be a no-consequence experience. There should be confidentiality between the student and PD so that the student knows she can be honest without her thoughts being used against her in any way. Also remember that some of the questions ask for the student to evaluate their Clinical Instructor. Honesty is important. If the student has concerns about the ability of the CI, the student should be able to express those concerns. The point of reflection is for students to learn how to conduct themselves as athletic trainers. There is no intention of the assignment being one that damages the relationship between the student and the CI. There is every intention of the assignment being one that causes critical evaluation. Because honest, thorough reflection has potential to be

Weekly Reflection Grading Rubric A

Assessment Criteria	Points
No weekly reflection or unacceptable reflection	0
Acceptable weekly reflection	1
Exceptional weekly reflection	2

Points will be included as part of the grade in your clinical course.

hurtful, I recommend that reflection be private. Only the scores should be shared with the clinical instructor.

Weekly Reflection Grading Rubric A is quick and easy to use. This allows the PD to provide quick feedback to many students.

The advantage of this rubric is that it is quick and easy to score and record a grade. When a program has many students completing reflections, this may be the rubric of choice. It is a good rubric for students getting in the habit of reflecting. The grader must define *unacceptable*, *acceptable*, and *exceptional*. Definitions of these terms may change, so students should be updated as needed. For example, *acceptable* first-year athletic training student reflections may not be *acceptable* senior athletic training student reflections. After *acceptable* and *unacceptable* are defined, there is very little ambiguity and thus there should be very little confusion about the rubric.

A second rubric can be used to assess student weekly reflections. Weekly Reflection Grading Rubric B is an expanded version of Rubric A. It provides a greater point spread for determining the quality of a reflection.

This rubric connects the reflection steps (recall, analysis, and synthesis) with grading criteria. This is a better rubric to use if one of the purposes of the assignment is to help students learn how to reflect. Professors have flexibility within Analysis and Synthesis to make quality judgments. Because it is easy to use and provides more detailed feedback to the students, this rubric may be preferred.

Sample Assignment #2 – Short Reflection Presentation

Make notes of reflections throughout the clinical rotation. The notes will not be turned in but organized to reflect as needed. You will present one learning experience to the class. The presentation will include a detailed explanation of what happened (recall), an explanation of apparent and extraneous events that influenced what happened (analysis), and an explanation of what was reinforced or learned and how this information will be used (synthesis). The presentation should be 10 to 15 minutes. (20 pts)

Many of our learning opportunities take place over several days and weeks, not a single day. Using daily reflections as our sole reflection activity causes

Weekly Reflection Grading Rubric B

Assessment Criteria	Points
Unacceptable reflection	0
Recall only	1
Analysis	2 – 3
Synthesis	4 – 5

Points will be included as part of the grade in your clinical course.

us to miss some learning opportunities. An assignment can span several days, weeks, or months to allow for a broader synthesis of information. The Short Reflection Presentation Assignment is suggested when one of the learning objectives of the program is helping students become comfortable with presenting information to a group. This assignment is good for students who need to get comfortable organizing and presenting material to others. Presenting information is a common task for athletic trainers. Coaches, athletes, administrators, and others must constantly be updated on policies, procedures, practices, expectations, etc.

The assignment can be completed several times throughout the semester for repeated presentation practice. Repeating presentations also allow the student to present different reflections and follows the learning over time teaching model used within athletic training.

Because an objective of this assignment is to help students become comfortable and competent with presentations, they should assess each other with this rubric. Grading each other stimulates critique and feedback of student's own work. If there is concern that students will be too easy on each other, then their name can be included on the grading rubric for the teacher to see or the teacher can count student peer scores as half the grade and the teacher score as the other half. In order to maintain confidentiality, peer evaluator scores and comments can be compiled onto a single sheet before being returned to the student. Notice very little weight is given to how the

---

Short Presentation Grading Rubric

Student _____   Date _____

	Poor					Excellent
Presenter's explanation of the events (recall)	0	1	2	3	4	5
Student explained the significance of the events as they relate to the practice of athletic training (analysis)	0	1	2	3	4	5
Student provided an explanation of what has been learned from the experience (synthesis)	0	1	2	3	4	5
Presentation was clear and logical	0	1	2	3	4	5

Total Points   _____

Strengths of the presentation:

Suggestions to improve the presentation:

information is presented. A student could use PowerPoint, but this assignment does not require such a formal presentation. The emphasis of the rubric is on the reflection steps and not on the mechanics of the presentation.

Sample Assignment #3 – Long Reflection Presentation

Make notes of reflections throughout a clinical assignment. The notes will not be turned in but will be organized and used as needed. You will then research their topic to compare and contrast their experience to the literature. You will make a professional presentation to the class that connects their experience to the knowledge presented in the literature. For example, if a student is presenting about effective communication techniques she should have an experience that serves as an example, and she should compare her experience with the literature. The presentation should include a detailed explanation of what happened (recall), an explanation of apparent and extraneous events that influenced what happened (analysis), and an explanation of what was reinforced or learned and how this information will be used (synthesis). If there is any sensitive information in the presentation, the student must hide the identity of those involved. The presentation should be 15 to 20 minutes. PowerPoint must be used. (50 pts)

The Long Reflection Presentation Assignment is ideal for advanced students who need to work on the specifics of a presentation. The formal presentation resembles one they would make at a professional conference and should be critiqued for both content and presentation mechanics. This assignment should be used to emphasize reflection, literature synthesis, and presentation mechanics. To do this assignment well students must do some research. Because of the many skills combined into a single assignment this exercise should be considered a capstone assignment.

The grading rubric is presented below. Notice the great detail of the rubric. Students should review the rubric thoroughly as they prepare their presentation.

This rubric is particular about the presentation itself. If the objective of the professor is to teach students how to make presentations, this rubric is more thorough in that regard. The scoring system can be adjusted to emphasize or de-emphasize a particular area.

Using this rubric shifts the objective of the assignment to teaching students how to present not reflect. Therefore, it should be used after students are proficient with reflection. Reflection allows the students to have a subject to talk about. Reflection also allows students to have a subject that is familiar to them and

potentially one that is beneficial to all. This rubric is the tool to help teach students how to develop and deliver a presentation. Boxes can be added or adjusted to the rubric to emphasize other areas. A teacher may want to emphasize the mechanics of developing PowerPoint and include criteria such as: appropriate number of words per slide, correct use of animation, etc. If an objective of the assignment is for the presenters to involve the class in discussion, then criteria related to student involvement would be appropriate. Adjustments can be made to the rubric as needed. As long as students have the rubric in advance, they should be able to match their presentation to the assessment criteria.

Sample Assignment #4 – Reflection Paper

Make notes of reflections throughout a clinical assignment. The notes will not be turned in but organized to use as needed. You will research a topic to compare and contrast personal experience to the literature. You will write a professional paper that shows synthesis of information. The paper should connect your experience to the knowledge presented in the literature. For example, if a student is presenting on effective communication techniques he should have an experience that serves as an example, and he should compare his experience to the literature. The paper is to include a detailed explanation of what happened (recall), an explanation of apparent and extraneous events that influenced what happened (analysis), and an explanation of what was reinforced or learned and how this information will be used (synthesis). If there is any sensitive information in the paper, the student must hide the identity of those involved. The paper must use sources both within and outside athletic training. References must be cited as per JAT formatting. The audience for the paper is other athletic training students. A draft of the paper will be turned in at midsemester for critique and editing by a classmate. The final paper is due at the end of the semester. See the accompanying grading rubric for specific assessment criteria. (50 pts)

Communication is paramount to the success of an athletic trainer, with written communication skills being just as important as verbal communication skills. We do not all have to like writing letters and papers, but we will have some minimal job requirements of communicating through writing. This assignment uses reflection as the knowledge gathering process and a paper as the synthesis process of that information.

A common education objective is to improve students' ability to organize and articulate thoughts and ideas. Papers are a good tool to determine how well our students can organize and express ideas

Oral Presentation Grading Rubric

Presenter _____   Topic _____

Evaluator _____   Date _____

	1–2	3–4	5–6	7–8	Score
Organization	Audience could not understand presentation because there was no sequence of information.	Audience had difficulty following presentation because student jumped around.	Student presented information in logical sequence.	Student presented information in logical, interesting sequence that audience could follow.	
Reflection Process	Student did not follow the reflection process.	Student recalled information but did not analyze or synthesize information well.	Student recalled and analyzed information but did not synthesize information well.	Student recalled, analyzed and synthesized information very well.	
Visual Aids	Student used unrelated or no visual aids.	Student occasionally used visual aids that only vaguely supported the presentation.	Student's visual aids related to the presentation.	Student's visual aids explained and reinforced the presentation.	
Mechanics	Presentation had four or more spelling errors and/or grammatical errors.	Presentation had three misspellings and/or grammatical errors.	Presentation had no more than two misspellings and/or grammatical errors.	Presentation had no misspellings or grammatical errors.	
Eye Contact	Student read the report with no eye contact.	Student occasionally used eye contact but read most of the report.	Student maintained eye contact most of the time but frequently returned to notes or slides.	Student maintained eye contact with the audience, seldom returning to notes or slides.	
Articulation	Student mumbled, incorrectly pronouncing terms, and spoke too quickly for students in the back of the class to hear.	Student's voice was low. Student incorrectly pronounced terms. Audience had difficulty hearing presentation.	Student's voice was clear. Student pronounced most words correctly. The audience heard the presentation.	Student used a clear voice and correct, precise pronunciation of terms. The audience heard the presentation.	
Time	Too short = 0	Too long = 1	Just right = 2		
				Total points	

Strengths of the presentation:

Suggestions to improve the presentation:

with smooth transitions and appropriate grouping of ideas. Reflection can provide the material, and a paper can reveal students' ability to convey what they have learned. This paper should be easy in that the students are relaying what they experienced. It will be harder when they attempt to organize it and teach us what they learned in their experience.

This assignment requires the use of multiple sources to write a paper. The requirements guide the student to writing a well-planned paper. Like the presentation assignment above, this is an advanced assignment that is best for an advanced student.

The strength of this grading rubric is that it is both tied to the reflection process and thorough in what it expects in the written paper. As an initial check students can critique their paper or a peer's paper against the criteria presented in the rubric. Peer review improves the overall quality of the final paper because students play the role of teacher and critically evaluate the paper.

Goals of Rubrics

The assignments presented in this chapter are designed to provide a chance for students to reflect while satisfying other course objectives. Rubrics provide the criteria to assess student learning. Together, assignments and rubrics provide a means of critiquing student reflections. This chapter should help students to be better critics of their own reflection. With this in mind, caution about grading rubrics needs to be expressed. Rubrics prompt students into writing what the teacher wants or expects to see. In doing so, rubrics help to mold behavior. The point of reflection is to allow students to indicate what they have learned from their own experience. Rubrics may stifle students' expressions rather than properly molding expressions. If the rubrics presented in this chapter create problems, discard them in favor of rubrics that allow teachers to assess student work while allowing students to express themselves openly.

Reflection Paper Grading Rubric

		Points Awarded		
	0	1	2	3
SKILLS & COMPETENCIES TO BE DEMONSTRATED				
Recall				
Uses athletic training terminology correctly				
Includes appropriate amount of detail				
Uses examples to support point				
Analysis				
Shows understanding of the profession of Athletic Training				
Thoughtfully analyzes experiences				
Objectively follows where evidence and reason lead				
Uses reasoning and evidence to reach conclusions				
Supports conclusions with clear cogent arguments				
Synthesis				
Integrates different perspectives/opinions				
Demonstrates originality of thought or approach				
Assembles pieces to form a coherent whole (synthesis)				
Brings together disparate elements to create new patterns				
Mechanics				
Free of spelling errors				
Free of punctuation and grammatical errors				
Clarity of presentation: smooth, easy to read				
Organization: logical sequence, arguments tied together				
Appropriate citation and reference format				

Comments

Athletic Training Educational Competencies

CHAPTER 4

Foundational Behaviors of Professional Practice

The best part of athletic training is working with people. The hardest part of athletic training is working with people.

Professional Behaviors

Athletic training is a people profession. As such we have an expectation about how we should deal with people. The expectations we have as professionals are integrated into this chapter. As with any profession we have guidance from multiple sources. Guidance for professional behavior comes primarily from our professional organization (e.g., National Athletic Trainers' Association [NATA] Code of Ethics) but also from the government (e.g., state practice acts). This chapter does not contain skills but rather helps the student put into action the foundational behaviors of athletic training. The primary objective of this chapter is to show the student how athletic training foundational behaviors influence the daily life of an athletic trainer.

Background Knowledge

In order for students to maximize their professional growth in this content area they must be:

1. Able to define professionalism.
2. Cognizant of cultural differences that affect patient care.
3. Familiar with the roles and responsibilities of health care professionals.
4. Familiar with the guidelines presented in: state laws, NATA Code of Ethics, Board of Certification (BOC) Standards of Practice, Health Insurance Portability and Accountability Act (HIPAA), Family Educational Rights and Privacy Act (FERPA), Role Delineation Study, policy and procedures manual, Occupational Safety and Health Administration (OSHA).

You can get more information at the following web pages:

NATA – National Athletic Trainers' Association at http://www.nata.org

BOC – Board of Certification at http://www.bocatc.org

HIPAA – US Department of Health and Human Services at http://www.hhs.gov.ocr/hipaa

FERPA – US Department of Education at http://www.ed.gov, search for FERPA

OSHA – US Department of Labor at http://www.osha.gov

CAATE – Commission on Accreditation of Athletic Training at http://www.caate.net

Goals

Write your goals that correspond to the content of this chapter.

Goal #	Goal

Discussion between the Student and ACI/CI

1. How does the state law define the scope of athletic training practice?

_____

_____

_____

_____

_____

2. Discuss a scenario in which multiple professionals were involved with the health care of a single patient. Describe each professional's role, responsibilities, and limitations of care.

_____

_____

_____

_____

_____

3. Do you know of any situations in which an AT violated or was accused of violating the NATA Code of Ethics? BOC Standard of Practice? State law?

_____

_____

_____

_____

_____

4. Are you familiar with any situation in which cultural differences prevented or could have prevented a patient from receiving optimal care?

_____

_____

_____

_____

5. Has your clinical instructor ever felt hopeless, discouraged, or burnt-out? How did he/she deal with it?

_____

_____

_____

_____

6. What does your clinical instructor like and not like about his/her job? Is your opinion the same concerning the positives and negatives of the job?

_____

_____

_____

_____

_____

7. What does your CI do to stay current in AT?

_____

_____

_____

_____

_____

Reflection

1. Describe a situation in which the patient needed you to be his/her advocate. In what way did you assist the patient?

_____

_____

_____

_____

_____

2. Describe a situation in which an AT demonstrated great/unusual integrity. Will you be able to act as this AT acted?

_____

_____

_____

_____

_____

3. Describe a situation in which an AT demonstrated unusual compassion for a patient. Would you be able to demonstrate the same level of compassion?

_____

_____

_____

_____

_____

4. Describe a situation in which an AT demonstrated effective communication skills. What do you need to do/learn in order to communicate as effectively as this AT?

_____

_____

_____

_____

_____

5. Describe a situation in which the AT did not involve the patient to the appropriate extent when designing a treatment plan. How could the situation have been improved?

_____

_____

_____

_____

_____

6. Describe your ideal job.

_____

_____

_____

_____

_____

7. What is one thing you have learned from your clinical instructor that you intend to include in your professional repertoire?

_____

_____

_____

_____

_____

8. What qualities of this clinical instructor do you want to emulate? Do you think you can?

_____

_____

_____

_____

_____

9. What motivates you?

_____

_____

_____

10. What is it about athletic training that excites you?

_____

_____

_____

_____

_____

11. What is it about athletic training that you wish you could change?

_____

_____

_____

_____

_____

12. What are some challenges to your athletic training knowledge you have faced in the past?

_____

_____

_____

_____

_____

13. What are your strengths as a learner?

_____

_____

_____

_____

_____

14. What are your strengths as a people professional?

_____

_____

_____

_____

_____

15. What challenges do you face in working with people?

_____

_____

_____

_____

_____

16. Everyone makes mistakes. Describe one mistake that you have seen. It does not have to be a big mistake. If you were the person who made the mistake, what would you do to correct this mistake? What can you do to avoid this or similar mistakes in the future?

_____

_____

_____

_____

_____

17. With what type of a leader do you want to work? What questions will you ask during your interview to determine the leadership style of your supervisor?

_____

_____

_____

_____

_____

18. Did you communicate well in a particular situation? If you were to repeat this experience what would you do the same and what would you do differently?

_____

_____

_____

_____

_____

19. What behaviors have you seen by ATs, coaches, patients, etc. that have facilitated good communication?

_____

_____

_____

_____

20. What behaviors have you seen by ATs, coaches, patients, etc. that have prevented good communication?

_____

_____

_____

_____

21. Emotion can interfere with the communication process. Explain a situation in which a person's emotion interfered with him/her delivering or receiving information.

_____

_____

_____

_____

_____

Skills To Be Assessed

None

Challenge Assignments

1. Summarize your state law.
2. What is the consequence of violating the NATA Code of Ethics?
3. Write a scenario in which an athletic trainer faces a conflict of interest.
4. Find each of the documents listed in Background Knowledge.
5. Find the mission statement of the NATA, BOC, Commission on Accreditation of Athletic Training Education (CAATE), Journal of Athletic Training, and Athletic Training Education Journal.
6. Describe your ideal Athletic Trainer.
7. Write a letter to the principal, Head ATC, Dean, etc. praising your clinical instructor. Be specific in explaining what he/she does well.

Journaling

Summarize the real-life Foundational Behaviors of Professional Practice experiences you have had. How have they helped your professional growth?

Date	CI/Rotation	Experience

Date	CI/Rotation	Experience

CHAPTER 5

Risk Management and Injury Prevention

Plan to prevent pathologies. Prepare to manage those that occur.

Injury Prevention

Participation in physical activity is accompanied by risk of injury. There is no way of preventing all injuries; however, common and foreseeable injuries should be minimized as much as possible. As a health care professional working with active individuals, the athletic trainer has a responsibility to minimize injury risk factors. The objective of this chapter is to provide the opportunity for students and CIs to determine the student's knowledge and skill in risk management and injury prevention. At the completion of this chapter the student should have a good understanding of the knowledge base needed in order to prevent injuries.

Background Knowledge

In order for students to maximize their professional growth in this content area they must be able to:

1. Recall risk factors for overuse injuries.
2. Explain the etiology and treatment of heat illness.
3. Explain prevention and treatment strategies for Methicillin-Resistant Staphylococcus Aureus (MRSA).
4. Read and interpret urine color charts and specific gravity measurements.
5. Describe normal heat distribution methods.
6. Recall risk factors associated with congenital and acquired abnormalities.
7. Identify organizations that monitor equipment design and construction.

Goals

Write your goals that correspond to the content of this chapter.

Goal #	Goal

Discussion between the Student and ACI/CI

1. What is the best way to conduct pre-participation physical examinations?

   _____

   _____

   _____

   _____

   _____

2. How do you monitor hydration status of your athletes?

   _____

   _____

   _____

   _____

   _____

3. What is the CI's role in issuing and maintaining protective equipment?

   _____

   _____

   _____

   _____

   _____

4. What is the emergency action plan for this particular venue?

   _____

   _____

   _____

   _____

   _____

5. What is the policy regarding lightning and other hazardous weather conditions?

   _____

   _____

   _____

   _____

   _____

6. Do any of your athletes have heat illness risk factors?

   _____

   _____

   _____

   _____

   _____

Reflection

1. Describe a situation in which a football player was not wearing proper protective equipment. What will you do as the certified athletic trainer to deal with situations like this?

_____

_____

_____

_____

_____

2. Describe your CI's policy regarding prophylactic ankle taping. What will your policy be when you are an ATC?

_____

_____

_____

_____

_____

3. What did you see that confused you?

_____

_____

_____

_____

_____

4. Recall a taping/bracing scenario that went very well. Why did it go well? What will you do in subsequent situations to ensure they go well?

_____

_____

_____

_____

_____

5. Recall a taping/bracing scenario that did not go very well. What went wrong? What will you do in subsequent situations to ensure they go well?

_____

_____

_____

_____

_____

6. What did you learn today that seems to contradict what you learned from books or professors?

_____

_____

_____

_____

_____

7. Recall a situation that was unsafe. What did the athletic trainer do to correct the situation? Would you have done anything different?

_____

_____

_____

_____

_____

8. Explain a situation in which you fit protective equipment. Did you have the supplies/equipment you needed? Did you make any modifications? Were they appropriate? Did you do a good job?

_____

_____

_____

_____

_____

9. Do you have any patients who are prone to injury due to problems with flexibility, posture, or anatomical abnormalities? What will you do to minimize injury rate and severity for these people?

_____

_____

_____

_____

_____

10. Recall a successful experience you had in fabricating/modifying protective equipment. What did you learn?

_____

_____

_____

_____

_____

Skills To Be Practiced and Assessed

Vital Signs

Body Composition

Baseline Measurements

Splinting

Equipment Fitting

Taping

Elastic Wraps

Hydration Assessment

VITAL SIGNS

Learning Over Time – Verification Chart

Skill	Individual Skills	Simulation/Random	Integrated into AT
Airway/Breathing			
Circulation			
Bleeding			
Skin Temp and Color			
Blood Pressure			
Pulse Rate and Rhythm			
Respiratory Rate and Rhythm			
Pupils			

Observer/date

Scoring Rubrics on pages 248–249

BODY COMPOSITION

Learning Over Time – Verification Chart

Skill	Individual Skills	Simulation/Random	Integrated into AT
BMI			
Skin Fold			

Observer/date _____ _____ _____

Scoring Rubrics on pages 250–251

BASELINE MEASUREMENTS

Learning Over Time – Verification Chart

Skill	Individual Skills	Simulation/Random	Integrated into AT
Limb Girth			
Limb Length			
Vision			
Posture			
Flexibility			
Strength			

Observer/date _____ _____ _____

Scoring Rubrics on pages 252–253

SPLINTING

Learning Over Time – Verification Chart

Skill	Individual Skills	Simulation/Random	Integrated into AT
Ankle			
Knee			
Hip			
Shoulder			
Elbow			
Wrist			
Finger			

Observer/date _____   _____   _____

Scoring Rubrics on pages 254–255

EQUIPMENT FITTING

Learning Over Time – Verification Chart

Skill	Individual Skills	Simulation/Random	Integrated into AT
Helmet			
Shoulder Pads			
Footwear			
Mouth Guard			
Knee Brace			
Ankle Brace			

Observer/date   _____   _____   _____

Scoring Rubrics on pages 256–257

TAPING

Learning Over Time – Verification Chart

Skill	Individual Skills	Simulation/Random	Integrated into AT
Ankle #1			
Ankle #2			
Arch			
Lower Leg			
Toe			
Wrist			
Thumb			
Elbow			
Fingers			

Observer/date _____   _____   _____

Scoring Rubrics on pages 258–259

ELASTIC WRAPS

Learning Over Time – Verification Chart

Skill	Individual Skills	Simulation/Random	Integrated into AT
Ankle			
Ankle – Cloth wrap			
Knee			
Hamstrings			
Quadriceps			
Hip – Flexors			
Hip – Adductors			
Shoulder			
Elbow			

Observer/date _____   _____   _____

Scoring Rubrics on pages 260–261

HYDRATION ASSESSMENT

Learning Over Time – Verification Chart

Skill	Individual Skills	Simulation/Random	Integrated into AT
Sling Psychrometer			
Urine Analysis			
Refractometer			

Observer/date   _____   _____   _____

Scoring Rubrics on pages 262–263

Challenge Assignments

1. Design a detailed heat illness prevention program.
2. Design a policy to prevent the spread of Methicillin-Resistant Staphylococcus Aureus (MRSA).
3. Develop a pre-participation physical examination.
4. Find and discuss the NATA position statements regarding prevention and management of heat illness.
5. List the more common cancers and identify the warning signs of each.
6. Teach an underclass member something you learned from this unit.
7. Present a case study of one of your patients who needed a unique taping/padding procedure.
8. Develop a plan to teach all the coaching staff CPR and First Aid.
9. Teach the first-year students about heat illness prevention strategies.
10. Develop an injury prevention program for an athletic team. Focus on the common and foreseeable injuries.

Journaling

Summarize the real life Risk Management and Injury Prevention experiences you have had. How have they helped your professional growth?

Date	CI/Rotation	Experience

Date	CI/Rotation	Experience

Pathology of Injuries and Illnesses

Physiological reaction does not always equal patient reaction.

Progression of Pathology

One of the main challenges that any health care professional has is matching the treatment plan with a patient's physiological response to injury. Doing too much too soon interferes with healing. Doing too little too late does nothing to facilitate healing. In order to assist the healing process in an optimal manner the athletic trainer must have a thorough understanding of physiology and progression of pathology. This chapter is designed to provide the student with practical experience in dealing with the progression of pathology. At the conclusion of this chapter students should be confident in their knowledge and skill in determining appropriate treatment based on their assessment of the patient's stage of healing.

Background Knowledge

In order for students to maximize their professional growth in this content area they must be able to:

1. Explain the inflammatory response.
2. Explain the healing process of soft tissue and bone.
3. Design a treatment plan that complements the stages of healing.
4. List the signs of infection.

Goals

Write your goals that correspond to the content of this chapter.

Goal #	Goal

Discussion between the Student and ACI/CI

1. Choose one of your patients. In what stage of healing is he/she? How does this patient's healing influence your choice of treatment options?

_____

_____

_____

_____

_____

2. Choose one of your patients. What should be done to maximize his/her tissue healing?

_____

_____

_____

_____

_____

3. Choose one of your patients. What is the expected outcome of his/her injury?

_____

_____

_____

_____

_____

4. What criteria do you use to determine if rehabilitation can progress?

_____

_____

_____

_____

_____

5. Have you had a patient progress more quickly than you expected?

_____

_____

_____

_____

_____

6. Have you had a patient progress more slowly than expected? What slowed the healing process?

_____

_____

_____

_____

Reflection

1. What is something that you saw or heard about a treatment plan that confused you?

   _____

   _____

   _____

   _____

   _____

2. What did you learn today that seems to contradict what you learned from books or professors?

   _____

   _____

   _____

   _____

   _____

3. Describe an injury situation in which two patients with approximately the same injury reacted very differently. Why do you think the patients reacted differently?

   _____

   _____

   _____

   _____

   _____

4. Recall a situation in which a patient did not progress as expected. Were there any physiological factors that interfered with tissue healing?

   _____

   _____

   _____

   _____

   _____

5. Recall a situation in which an athlete's or coach's expectations for return to play were not realistic based on the healing that needed to occur.

   _____

   _____

   _____

   _____

   _____

Skills To Be Practiced and Assessed

Systemic Pathology Assessment Skills

SYSTEMIC PATHOLOGY ASSESSMENT SKILLS

Learning Over Time – Verification Chart

Skill	Individual Skills	Simulation/Random	Integrated into AT
Otoscope			
Ophthalmoscope			
Stethoscope			
Heart sounds			
Lung sounds			
Bowel sounds			

Observer/date   _____   _____   _____

Scoring Rubrics on pages 264–265

Challenge Assignments

1. Outline the healing process.
2. Make a chart of the expected healing times of a variety of injuries.
3. Explain how diabetes or other physiological problems influence the healing process.
4. Present a patient as a case study. Identify some exercises that are commonly used for such problems but are contraindicated for this particular patient. Explain why.
5. Make a list of pathologies that may not have to be fully healed in order to return an athlete to full activity. In your list also indicate how you will protect the athlete during his/her weakened state.
6. Make a list of injured patients during your rotation. Explain the healing status of each individual.
7. Explain how nutrition (poor and optimal) influences healing.

Journaling

Summarize the real-life Pathology of Injury and Illness experiences you have had. How have they helped your professional growth?

Date	CI/Rotation	Experience

Date	CI/Rotation	Experience

Orthopedic Clinical Examination and Diagnosis

Accurate diagnosis provides the foundation for accurate treatment.

Orthopedic Evaluation

A large percentage of the athletic trainer's patients suffer from orthopedic injuries. Proper management of sprains, strains, contusions, and fractures begins with proper diagnosis. Accurate diagnosis occurs as a result of proper clinical examination knowledge and skill. This chapter provides students with opportunities to practice their orthopedic evaluation skills and diagnostic decision making.

Background Knowledge

In order for students to maximize their professional growth in this content area they must be able to:

1. Identify anatomy, including bony and soft tissue landmarks, muscle attachments, and nerve innervations.
2. Identify normal physiology and pathophysiology.
3. Recall typical ranges of motion for each joint.
4. Assess isometric, concentric, and eccentric muscle strength.
5. Explain the etiology and treatment of common orthopedic pathologies (e.g., scoliosis, osteoarthritis, stress fractures, etc.).
6. Identify common acquired and congenital risk factors that predispose a patient to injury.

Goals

Write your goals that correspond to the content of this chapter.

Goal #	Goal

Discussion between the Student and ACI/CI

1. Have the CI choose a condition. The student should be able to explain the etiology, pathology, typical course of treatment, and approximate time for return to play.

   _____

   _____

   _____

   _____

   _____

2. Discuss signs and diagnostic tests for a variety of orthopedic conditions (e.g., spondylolysis, metatarsal stress fracture, glenohumeral dislocation, etc.)

   _____

   _____

   _____

   _____

   _____

3. What is the oddest injury you have seen?

   _____

   _____

   _____

   _____

   _____

4. What injuries do you commonly see with each sport?

   _____

   _____

   _____

   _____

   _____

5. What is the most serious injury you have seen?

   _____

   _____

   _____

   _____

   _____

6. What diagnostic imaging techniques do the team physicians prefer?

_____

_____

_____

_____

_____

Reflection

1. Reflect on an injury situation that did not progress as expected.

_____

_____

_____

_____

_____

2. What diagnostic skill/tool confused you?

_____

_____

_____

_____

_____

3. Recall an evaluation scenario that went very well. Why did it go well? What could be done in subsequent situations to ensure they also go well?

_____

_____

_____

_____

_____

4. Recall an injury evaluation scenario that did not go very well. What went wrong? What could be done in subsequent situations to ensure they go well?

_____

_____

_____

_____

_____

5. Perform a skill. Examples of skills you could choose are Lachman's test, shoulder apprehension test, and manual muscle test of the brachiialis. Analyze your skill. What did you do well? What do you need to practice?

_____

_____

_____

_____

_____

6. Recall an event where two people had different diagnoses of the same pathology. Explain how two people can have different explanations for the same pathology.

_____

_____

_____

_____

_____

7. What did you learn today that seems to contradict what you learned from books or professors?

_____

_____

_____

_____

_____

8. Reflect on the way your CI performs a diagnostic test that is different from how you perform a test.

_____

_____

_____

_____

_____

9. Recall a situation that initially appeared to be one pathology but turned out to be another pathology. Explain the difference.

_____

_____

_____

_____

_____

10. Describe a person who has very good diagnostic skills. What is it that makes them good?

_____

_____

_____

_____

Skills To Be Practiced and Assessed

Foot, Ankle, and Leg Evaluation

Knee and Thigh Evaluation

Hip Evaluation

Back and Neck Evaluation

Shoulder and Arm Evaluation

Elbow, Wrist, and Hand Evaluation

Head and Face Evaluation

FOOT, ANKLE, AND LEG EVALUATION

Learning Over Time – Verification Chart

Skill	Individual Skills	Simulation/Random	Integrated into AT
History/Subjective		History	
Observation		Observation	
Static Posture			
Dynamic Posture			
Deformity			
Palpation		Palpation	
Soft Tissue			
Bones and Landmarks			
ROM (Active and Passive)		ROM	
Toe – Flx & Ext			
Inversion			
Eversion			
Plantar Flexion			
Dorsiflexion			

Strength		Strength	
Toe Flx & Ext			
Inversion			
Eversion			
Plantar Flexion			
Dorsiflexion			
Special Tests		Special Tests	
Lat (ATF, CF, PTF)			
Med (Deltoid)			
Tendon			
Tib Fib Joint			
Great Toe MP			
Rule out Fracture			
Circ & Neurological		Circ & Neurological	
Skin Temp and Color			
Dermatomes			
Myotomes			
Reflexes			
Pulse			
Functional Activities		Functional Activities	

Observer/date   _____   _____   _____

Scoring Rubrics on pages 266–268

KNEE AND THIGH EVALUATION

Learning Over Time – Verification Chart

Skill	Individual Skills	Simulation/Random	Integrated into AT
History/Subjective		History/Subjective	
Observation		Observation	
Static Posture			
Dynamic Posture			
Deformity			
Palpation		Palpation	
Soft Tissue			
Bones & Landmarks			
ROM (Active & Passive)		ROM	
Flexion			
Extension			
Patella Mobility			
Strength		Strength	
Flexion			
Extension			
Special Tests		Special Tests	
ACL			

PCL			
MCL			
LCL			
Meniscus			
Iliotibial Band			
Patella Tests			
Femur (Stress Fx)			
Rule out Fracture			
Circ & Neurological		Circ & Neurological	
Skin Temp & Color			
Dermatomes			
Myotomes			
Reflexes			
Pulse			
Functional Activities		Functional Activities	

Observer/date   _____   _____   _____

Scoring Rubrics on pages 269–271

HIP EVALUATION

Learning Over Time – Verification Chart

Skill	Individual Skills	Simulation/Random	Integrated into AT
History/Subjective		History/Subjective	
Observation		Observation	
Static Posture			
Dynamic Posture			
Deformity			
Palpation		Palpation	
Soft Tissue			
Bones & Landmarks			
ROM (Active & Passive)		ROM	
Flexion			
Extension			
Abduction			
Adduction			
Rotation			
Strength		Strength	
Flexion			
Extension			

Abduction			
Adduction			
Circumduction			
Special Tests		Special Tests	
Pubofemoral Lig			
Iliofemoral Lig			
Ischiofemoral Lig			
Acetabulum			
Pubic Symphysis			
Rule out Fracture			
Circ & Neurological		Circ & Neurological	
Skin Temp & Color			
Dermatomes			
Myotomes			
Reflexes			
Pulse			
Functional Activities		Functional Activities	

Observer/date _____   _____   _____

Scoring Rubrics on pages 272–274

BACK AND NECK EVALUATION

Learning Over Time – Verification Chart

Skill	Individual Skills	Simulation/Random	Integrated into AT
History/Subjective		History/Subjective	
Observation		Observation	
Static Posture			
Dynamic Posture			
Deformity			
Palpation		Palpation	
Soft Tissue			
Bones & Landmarks			
ROM (Active & Passive)		ROM	
Flexion			
Extension			
Lateral Flexion			
Rotation			
Strength		Strength	
Flexion			
Extension			
Lateral Flexion			
Rotation			

Limb Strength			
Special Tests		Special Tests	
Sacroiliac Joint			
Facets			
Discs			
Intervertebral Foramen			
Rule out Fracture			
Circ & Neurological		Circ & Neurological	
Skin Temp & Color			
Dermatomes			
Myotomes			
Reflexes			
Pulse			
Functional Activities		Functional Activities	

Observer/date _____ _____ _____

Scoring Rubrics on pages 275–277

SHOULDER AND ARM EVALUATION

Learning Over Time – Verification Chart

Skill	Individual Skills	Simulation/Random	Integrated into AT
History/Subjective		History/Subjective	
Observation		Observation	
Static Posture			
Dynamic Posture			
Deformity			
Palpation		Palpation	
Soft Tissue			
Bones & Landmarks			
ROM (Active & Passive)		ROM	
Flexion/Extension			
Abduction/Adduction			
Internal/External Rotation			
Horizontal Abd & Add			
Circumduction			
Scapula Movements			
Strength		Strength	
Flexion/Extension			
Abduction/Adduction			

Internal/External Rotation			
Horizontal Abd & Add			
Scapula Protract & Retract			
Scapula Elevation			
Special Tests		Special Tests	
GH Stability			
Labrum			
Rotator Cuff			
Impingement			
Acromioclavicular Jt			
Sternoclavicular Jt			
Rule out Fracture			
Circ & Neurological		Circ & Neurological	
Skin Temp & Color			
Dermatomes			
Myotomes			
Reflexes			
Pulse			
Functional Activities		Functional Activities	

Observer/date _____   _____   _____

Scoring Rubrics on pages 278–281

ELBOW, WRIST, AND HAND EVALUATION

Learning Over Time – Verification Chart

Skill	Individual Skills	Simulation/Random	Integrated into AT
History/Subjective		History/Subjective	
Observation		Observation	
Static Posture			
Dynamic Posture			
Deformity			
Palpation		Palpation	
Soft Tissue			
Bones & Landmarks			
ROM (Active & Passive)		ROM	
Elbow Flexion/Extension			
Pronation/Supination			
Wrist Flexion/Extension			
Thumb Movements			
Finger Movements			
Strength		Strength	
Elbow Flexion/Extension			
Pronation/Supination			
Wrist Flexion/Extension			

Thumb Movements			
Finger Movements			
Special Tests		Special Tests	
Elbow MCL			
Elbow LCL			
Annular Lig			
Med & Lat Epicondylitis			
Wrist Stability			
Wrist TFCC			
Thumb Joints & Bones			
Finger Joints & Bones			
Rule out Fractures			
Circ & Neurological		Circ & Neurological	
Skin Temp & Color			
Dermatomes			
Myotomes			
Reflexes			
Pulse			
Functional Activities		Functional Activities	

Observer/date _____   _____   _____

Scoring Rubrics on pages 282–284

HEAD AND FACE EVALUATION

Learning Over Time – Verification Chart

Skill	Individual Skills	Simulation/Random	Integrated into AT
History/Subjective		History/Subjective	
Observation		Observation	
CSF			
Deformity			
Palpation			
Deformity			
Signs/Symptoms		Signs/Symptoms	
LOC			
Headache			
Concentration			
Coordination			
ST Memory			
LT Memory			
Eye Function			

Cranial Nerve Assessment		Cranial Nerve Assessment	
Home Instructions		Home Instructions	
Emergency Protocols			

Observer/date _____ _____ _____

Scoring Rubrics on pages 285–287

Challenge Assignments

1. Recall an evaluation test or technique you have used recently. What evidence exists of its reliability and validity?
2. Make a list of pathologies in the left column and their differential diagnoses in the right column.
3. Evaluate five patients. Discuss your assessment with your clinical instructor.
4. Review the files of five patients. Are there any notes about diagnoses that you do not understand?
5. Make a list of the special tests for each body part. List the primary anatomical structure the test is intended to stress. List secondary anatomical structures that could be stressed by this test.
6. What injuries are common in high school athletes that are not common in college and professional athletes?
7. List all the possible questions you could ask a patient to obtain a thorough history for an acute injury. List all the possible questions for a chronic injury as well.

Journaling

Summarize the real-life Orthopedic Clinical Examination and Diagnosis experiences you have had. How have they helped your professional growth?

Date	CI/Rotation	Experience

Date	CI/Rotation	Experience

Medical Conditions and Disabilities

Athletes are people. People have a variety of medical conditions.

Medical Conditions and Physical Activity

As health care providers to physically active individuals, athletic trainers manage disorders that are non-orthopedic in nature. Patients may present with conditions such as asthma or diabetes. While physical activity likely did not cause these conditions, the AT must still have a thorough working knowledge of a variety of medical conditions. The AT may or may not be in a position of diagnosis but he/she will be in a position to play a role in managing the condition, particularly as the condition relates to and influences physical activity. Because of this it is important that the AT have a good working knowledge of how a variety of medical conditions affect physical activity. It is equally important to understand how physical activity influences a variety of medical conditions. The purpose of this chapter is to provide opportunities to practice skills and knowledge that assist in the diagnosis and management of several medical conditions and disabilities.

Background Knowledge

In order for students to maximize their professional growth in this content area they must be able to:

1. List the effects of age, diabetes, dehydration, chronic disease, etc. on tissue healing.
2. Identify the signs and symptoms of diabetes, insulin shock, diabetic coma, and other medical conditions.
3. Utilize a thorough working knowledge of anatomy and physiology of the body systems (i.e., skeletal, endocrine, nervous, digestive, muscular, integumentary, circulatory, lymphatic, respiratory, reproductive).
4. List common disorders of each of the body systems.

Goals

Write your goals that correspond to the content of this chapter.

Goal #	Goal

Discussion between the Student and ACI/CI

1. Have the CI choose a condition. The student should be able to explain the etiology, pathology, typical course of treatment, and approximate time for return to play. Sample conditions include strep throat, mononucleosis, asthma, hypertrophic cardiomyopathy, etc.

   _____

   _____

   _____

   _____

   _____

2. With what odd/interesting medical conditions has the CI dealt?

   _____

   _____

   _____

   _____

   _____

3. Are there any common conditions you see with your group of athletes?

   _____

   _____

   _____

   _____

   _____

4. Do you feel prepared to handle all medical conditions that may come your way?

   _____

   _____

   _____

   _____

   _____

5. What guidelines do you use to determine when to refer a patient to a physician?

   _____

   _____

   _____

   _____

   _____

6. To which physicians are different illnesses referred?

_____

_____

_____

_____

_____

7. Have you ever had an athlete experience an adverse reaction to medicine?

_____

_____

_____

_____

_____

Reflection

1. What is something you saw regarding general medical conditions that confused you?

_____

_____

_____

_____

_____

2. Describe a minor medical condition that has potential to be a big problem.

_____

_____

_____

_____

_____

3. What did you learn today that seems to contradict what you learned from books or professors?

_____

_____

_____

_____

_____

4. What policies do you plan to implement to ensure that all general medical conditions are handled properly?

_____

_____

_____

_____

_____

Skills To Be Practiced and Assessed

Peak Flow Meter

Body Temperature

Pupil Reaction

Urinalysis

Abdominal Palpation

Throat/Neck Palpation

MEDICAL CONDITIONS AND DISABILITIES

Learning Over Time – Verification Chart

Skills	Individual skills	Simulation/Random	Integrated into AT
Peak flow meter			
Body temperature			
Pupil reaction			
Urinalysis			
Abdominal palpation		Palpations	
Liver			
Spleen			
Appendix			
Throat/Neck palpation			
Lymph nodes			

Observer/date   _____   _____   _____

Scoring Rubrics on pages 288–289

Challenge Assignments

1. Make a table with common illnesses in the first column and common signs and symptoms across the top row. Fill in the table with x's to indicate that the sign or symptom matches the pathology. Make a different table for each body system.
2. Make a list of common illnesses and differential diagnoses.
3. Make a table with common illnesses in the first column and common diagnostic tests across the top row. Fill in the table with x's to indicate that the test is typically used to help diagnose the pathology. Make a different table for each body system.
4. Choose five different systemic pathologies. Teach a younger student about the pathologies. In your explanation be sure to indicate: etiology, signs/symptoms, diagnostic tests, typical treatment plan, and effect on athletic participation.
5. Take a thorough history on an individual with a skin disorder.

Journaling

Summarize the real-life Medical Conditions and Disabilities experiences you have had. How have they helped your professional growth?

Date	CI/Rotation	Experience

Date	CI/Rotation	Experience

CHAPTER 9

Acute Care of Injuries and Illnesses

A calm, confident voice is the most important emergency management tool.

Acute Care

Athletic Trainers must be ready at any moment to provide acute care for injury or illness. The pathology may be as benign as a contusion or it may be as serious as life-threatening heat stroke. The athletic trainer rarely gets a warning that an emergency is going to happen. He/she is forced by the situation to immediately recall and practice lifesaving skills. While most acute injuries are not emergencies, the athletic trainer must always be prepared for all levels of severity in injuries. The purpose of this chapter is to review the knowledge and skill necessary to properly manage acute injuries that range from minor to life-threatening.

Background Knowledge

In order for students to maximize their professional growth in this content area they must be able to:

1. Perform CPR.
2. Identify the signs and symptoms of internal bleeding, inflammation, concussion, cervical injury.
3. Explain the function of all cranial nerves.
4. Employ universal precautions.
5. Recognize and manage shock, diabetic coma, seizure, drug overdose, allergic reaction.
6. Recall modes of transmission, typical treatments, typical signs and symptoms of common systemic pathologies.
7. Recognize and manage cardiac and pulmonary emergencies.

Goals

Write your goals that correspond to the content of this chapter.

Goal #	Goal

Discussion between the Student and ACI/CI

1. Discuss emergency situations with which you have been involved.

   _____

   _____

   _____

   _____

   _____

2. What pathologies might exist if the patient presents with the following signs/symptoms?

   Skin is moist _____

   Skin is cold _____

   Pupils are unresponsive to light _____

   Patient complains of loss of function _____

3. Have you ever performed CPR? What was the situation? What did you learn from this experience?

   _____

   _____

   _____

   _____

   _____

4. What policy(ies) help prevent the spread of communicable diseases?

   _____

   _____

   _____

   _____

   _____

5. How do you know when to refer a patient for head, neck, thoracic, arm, leg, low back, hip injury?

   _____

   _____

   _____

   _____

   _____

6. Have you ever been too cautious in referring patients?

   _____

   _____

   _____

   _____

7. Have you ever had a situation in which you wish you would have been quicker to refer a patient to a physician?

_____

_____

_____

_____

_____

8. What criteria do you use to determine emergency versus nonemergency situations?

_____

_____

_____

_____

_____

9. What home instructions do you give following a head injury?

_____

_____

_____

_____

_____

10. What home instructions do you give following an ankle sprain?

_____

_____

_____

_____

_____

11. Discuss all participants' roles in spine boarding and transporting an injured athlete.

_____

_____

_____

_____

_____

12. Have you ever treated an athlete with a neck injury? What happened?

_____

_____

_____

_____

13. What is your Emergency Action Plan?

_____

_____

_____

_____

_____

Reflection

1. Recall an open wound. What factors interfered with optimal management?

_____

_____

_____

_____

_____

2. Revisit a situation in which an athlete suffered from a local infection. Could this infection have been prevented?

_____

_____

_____

_____

_____

3. What is something that you saw that confused you?

_____

_____

_____

_____

_____

4. Recall an injury management scenario that went very well. Why did it go well? What will you do in subsequent situations to ensure they go well?

_____

_____

_____

_____

_____

5. Recall an emergency scenario that went very well. Why did it go well? What will you do in subsequent situations to ensure they go well?

_____

_____

_____

_____

_____

6. Recall an injury management scenario that did not go very well. What went wrong? What will you do in subsequent situations to ensure they go well?

_____

_____

_____

_____

_____

7. Recall an emergency scenario that did not go very well. What went wrong? What will you do in subsequent situations to ensure they go well?

_____

_____

_____

_____

_____

8. What did you learn today that seems to contradict what you learned from books or professors?

_____

_____

_____

_____

_____

9. If someone had a myocardial infarction today would you be prepared to handle the situation? How do you know?

_____

_____

_____

_____

_____

10. Have you ever used knowledge or skills that you did not expect to use as an AT?

_____

_____

_____

_____

_____

Skills To Be Practiced and Assessed

Level of Consciousness

Rescue Breathing

CPR

AED

Assessing Breathing, Circulation, Body Temperature

Removing Face mask

Patient Transport

Open Wound Management

Controlling Bleeding

Immobilization

Crutch Fitting

EMERGENCY MANAGEMENT

Learning Over Time – Verification Chart

Skill	Individual Skills	Simulation/Random	Integrated into AT
Level of consciousness			
Rescue breathing			
CPR			
AED			
Assess breathing status			
Assess circulation			
Assess body temperature			
Remove face mask			
Patient transport			
Open wound treatment			
Control bleeding			

Observer/date _____   _____   _____

Scoring Rubrics on pages 290–291

IMMOBILIZATION AND CRUTCH FITTING

Learning Over Time – Verification Chart

Skill	Individual Skills	Simulation/Random	Integrated into AT
Ankle			
Knee			
Hip			
Shoulder			
Elbow			
Wrist/Hand			
Spine			
Crutch Fitting			

Observer/date   _____   _____   _____

Scoring Rubrics on pages 292–293

Challenge Assignments

1. Draw the brachial plexus, sacral plexus, and lumbar plexus.
2. Compare and contrast three different concussion classification systems.
3. Review the emergency action plan (EAP) for your clinical site. Do you know of any emergency situations that are not covered by the plan?
4. Instruct an athlete on home care following a concussion.
5. Describe an emergency situation that occurred during your clinical assignment. Could you have handled the situation? What will you do to prepare for similar emergencies in the future?
6. Make a quick reference notebook of the signs/symptoms and treatment of the following pathologies: closed head trauma, heat illness, cold illness, seizure, acute asthma attack, shock, internal hemorrhage, peripheral nerve injuries, diabetic coma, insulin shock, drug overdose, allergic reaction.

Journaling

Summarize the real-life Acute Care of Injury and Illness experiences you have had. How have they helped your professional growth?

Date	CI/Rotation	Experience

Date	CI/Rotation	Experience

CHAPTER 10

Therapeutic Modalities

A match between the effect of the modality and the body's physiological response produces the desired treatment outcome.

Therapeutic Modalities

Athletic trainers use a variety of tools in an attempt to facilitate an optimal healing environment. Modalities assist with managing pain, limiting secondary injury, and promoting healing. Each application or series of applications is designed to satisfy a physiological goal. With a thorough knowledge of desired and undesirable outcomes the athletic trainer can prescribe, administer, and adjust modality settings as necessary. The purpose of this chapter is to provide students with an opportunity to administer and adjust modalities to match patient treatment goals.

Background Knowledge

In order for students to maximize their professional growth in this content area they must be able to:

1. List indications and contraindications for use of each modality.
2. Select alternatives for each modality.
3. List the criteria for determining when to discontinue or increase the intensity, time, and other aspects of a modality.
4. List desired and undesirable outcomes of each modality.
5. Explain the basis for selecting modality parameters.
6. Record a modality application so another professional can duplicate your application.
7. Relate treatment goals to modality selection.
8. Explain the stages of wound/tissue healing.

Goals

Write your goals that correspond to the content of this chapter.

Goal #	Goal

Discussion between the Student and ACI/CI

1. What setup parameters do you use for _____? (Provide as much detail as possible so the answer can be specific.)

_____

_____

_____

_____

_____

2. Are there any modalities that you particularly like or do not like using? Why?

_____

_____

_____

_____

_____

3. What is your philosophy on modality use?

_____

_____

_____

_____

_____

4. Have you had a situation in which a patient adversely responded to a modality treatment?

_____

_____

_____

_____

_____

5. If money was no concern, what modalities would you purchase?

_____

_____

_____

_____

_____

Reflection

1. Explain a situation in which a modality played a large role in an athlete's return to play.

   _____

   _____

   _____

   _____

   _____

2. Explain a situation in which the person did not respond to a modality treatment in the way you expected. Provide explanations for why this happened.

   _____

   _____

   _____

   _____

   _____

3. What is something you saw that confused you?

   _____

   _____

   _____

   _____

   _____

4. Recall a situation in which you administered the initial modality treatment to a patient. Did you communicate well with the patient? What is the evidence that you did or did not communicate well with the patient?

   _____

   _____

   _____

   _____

   _____

5. Extraneous variables interfere with our actions/decisions. For example, you may want to refer a patient to a specific physician, but insurance may not pay for services from this physician. Recall a situation in which extraneous circumstances caused your CI to administer a modality different from the usual administration.

   _____

   _____

   _____

   _____

6. What did you learn today that seems to contradict what you learned from books or professors?

_____

_____

_____

_____

_____

Skills To Be Practiced and Assessed

Cryotherapy

Thermotherapy

Contrast Therapy

Diathermy

Electrical Stimulation

Therapeutic Ultrasound

Traction

Massage

Intermittent Compression

Biofeedback

MODALITY APPLICATION

Learning Over Time – Verification Chart

Skills	Individual Skills	Simulation/Random	Integrated into AT
Infrared modality		**Infrared modality**	
Cryotherapy			
Ice packs			
Ice massage			
Chemical cold packs			
Vapocoolant spray			
Ice immersion			
Thermotherapy			
Moist heat packs			
Whirlpool baths			
Paraffin baths			
Contrast Therapy			
Diathermy			
Electrical stimulation		**Electrical stimulation**	
Direct Current			

Iontophoresis			
For pain control			
For muscle contraction			
Therapeutic ultrasound		**Therapeutic ultrasound**	
Pulsed US			
Continuous US			
Phonophoresis			
Traction		**Traction**	
Cervical			
Lumbar			
Massage		**Massage**	
Intermittent Compression		**Intermittent Compression**	
Biofeedback		**Biofeedback**	

Observer/date _____ _____ _____

Scoring Rubrics on pages 294–296

Challenge Assignments

1. Choose an injury scenario from your clinical experience in which modalities were used. Describe how the modalities interacted with the healing process.
2. Choose an injury situation from your clinical experience in which modalities were not used. Assuming you had any modalities you desired, select the appropriate modalities and treatment parameters for this situation.
3. Review the literature for the effectiveness of each modality you have used.
4. Recall a modality you have used recently. What evidence do you have that the modality accomplished your objective?
5. Teach an underclass student how to apply a modality.
6. Make a list of indications and contraindications for all modalities at your clinical education site.
7. Draw a diagram for the controls used to set parameters of the electrical modalities.
8. Make a check-off sheet for all you would do for a modality treatment. Be sure to include setup/preparation, education of patient, use, and cleanup.

Journaling

Summarize the real-life experiences you have had that require administration of Therapeutic Modalities. How have they helped your professional growth?

Date	CI/Rotation	Experience

Date	CI/Rotation	Experience

Conditioning and Rehabilitative Exercise

Tissue responds to the demands placed upon it. The challenge is to provide the appropriate stress to achieve desired results.

Tissue Healing and Reconditioning

Injured tissue heals in response to the demands placed upon it. Stress which is too great interferes with the healing process. Stress which is too minimal fails to stimulate the tissue maturation process. In managing pathologies the athletic trainer is responsible for assessing tissue healing status and providing appropriate stress to optimize healing. The objective of the reconditioning process is to provide optimal stress to optimize healing. This chapter provides students with the opportunity to utilize their knowledge of tissue healing and to practice skills that assist in reconditioning injured patients.

Background Knowledge

In order for students to maximize their professional growth in this content area they must be able to:

1. Identify typical ROM for each joint (see Chapter 22).
2. Perform measurements of strength, endurance, speed, and power.
3. Identify means of improving balance, neuromuscular control, coordination, agility, and cardiorespiratory endurance.
4. Identify factors that positively or negatively influence wound healing.

5. Explain stages of wound/tissue healing.
6. Recall typical timelines for healing fractures, sprains, strains, and contusions.
7. Classify the playing status of an athlete with fracture, sprain, strain, contusion.
8. Explain common surgical techniques.
9. Explain and demonstrate common therapeutic exercises.
10. List the physiological effects of immobilization.
11. Describe adaptations of acute and chronic exercise.
12. Explain indications and contraindications for each exercise.
13. Explain and demonstrate common strength training exercises—squat, heel raises, power clean, bench press, shoulder press, dead lift, arm curl, triceps extension, leg curl, knee extension, leg press, lunge.
14. Establish rehabilitation goals based on diagnosis and athletic activity.
15. List the indications and contraindications for exercises.
16. Incorporate a variety of techniques/equipment into the rehab program e.g., aquatic rehab, stationary bike, exercise balls, treadmill, balance equipment, reaction drills, neuromuscular control exercises, functional activities.
17. Explain the psychological aspects of rehabilitation.

Goals

Write your goals that correspond to the content of this chapter.

Goal #	Goal

Discussion between the Student and ACI/CI

1. What is your philosophy of rehabilitation?

   _____

   _____

   _____

   _____

   _____

2. What do you do to motivate the unmotivated patient?

   _____

   _____

   _____

   _____

   _____

3. What do you do to limit the eager patient?

   _____

   _____

   _____

   _____

   _____

4. What has been a difficult rehabilitation case? Why?

   _____

   _____

   _____

   _____

   _____

5. What exercises do you like for rotator cuff pathology? Why?

   _____

   _____

   _____

   _____

   _____

6. What exercises do you like for strengthening the vastus medialis oblique VMO? Why?

   _____

   _____

   _____

   _____

7. What exercises do you include in rehab that other people typically do not include?

_____

_____

_____

_____

_____

8. Have you had an athlete with unique anatomy (e.g., extreme hip retroversion) that presented challenges to rehabilitation?

_____

_____

_____

_____

_____

9. Have you had a post-surgical rehabilitation that was particularly challenging? What made it challenging?

_____

_____

_____

_____

_____

10. How do you determine that a person is ready to return to full activity?

_____

_____

_____

_____

_____

Reflection

1. Revisit a rehabilitation program that went very well. Why did it go so well? What will you do in subsequent situations to ensure they go well?

_____

_____

_____

_____

2. Revisit a rehabilitation program that did not go very well. Why did it not go well?

_____

_____

_____

_____

3. Recall an exercise that your CI used that you did not know. Are there other versions of this exercise you could incorporate into your therapeutic exercise repertoire?

_____

_____

_____

_____

_____

4. What is something that you saw that confused you?

_____

_____

_____

_____

_____

5. Recall one rehabilitation exercise you instructed. Did you communicate well with the patient? What is the evidence that you did or did not communicate well with the patient?

_____

_____

_____

_____

_____

6. Extraneous variables interfere with our actions/decisions. For example, you may want to refer a patient to a specific physician, but insurance may not pay for services from this person. Recall a situation in which extraneous circumstances caused your CI to do something different than what he/she wanted to do. Was there any way to predict and avoid the problems caused by these extraneous variables?

_____

_____

_____

_____

7. What did you learn today that seems to contradict what you learned from books or professors?

_____

_____

_____

_____

Skills To Be Practiced and Assessed

Therapeutic Exercises for:

Foot, Ankle and Lower Leg

Knee and Thigh

Hip

Back and Neck

Shoulder

Arm and Elbow

Hand and Wrist

Joint Mobilization

Aquatic Therapy

PNF

Power, Agility, Speed, Endurance

THERAPEUTIC EXERCISE – FOOT, ANKLE, LOWER LEG

Learning Over Time – Verification Chart

Skills	Individual Skills	Simulation/Random	Integrated into AT
Range of Motion		Range of Motion	
Strength		Strength	
Coordination/NM control		Coordination/NM control	
Functional/Sport Specific		Functional/Sport Specific	

Observer/date _____ _____ _____

Scoring Rubrics on pages 297–298

THERAPEUTIC EXERCISE – KNEE AND THIGH

Learning Over Time – Verification Chart

Skills	Individual Skills	Simulation/Random	Integrated into AT
Range of Motion		Range of Motion	
Strength		Strength	
Coordination/NM control		Coordination/NM control	
Functional/Sport Specific		Functional/Sport Specific	

Observer/date _____   _____   _____

Scoring Rubrics on pages 299–300

THERAPEUTIC EXERCISE – HIP

Learning Over Time – Verification Chart

Skills	Individual Skills	Simulation/Random	Integrated into AT
Range of Motion		Range of Motion	
Strength		Strength	
Coordination/NM control		Coordination/NM control	
Functional/Sport Specific		Functional/Sport Specific	

Observer/date   _____   _____   _____

Scoring Rubrics on pages 301–302

THERAPEUTIC EXERCISE – BACK AND NECK

Learning Over Time – Verification Chart

Skills	Individual Skills	Simulation/Random	Integrated into AT
Range of Motion		Range of Motion	
Strength		Strength	
Coordination/NM control		Coordination/NM control	
Functional/Sport Specific		Functional/Sport Specific	

Observer/date _____ _____ _____

Scoring Rubrics on pages 303–304

THERAPEUTIC EXERCISE – SHOULDER

Learning Over Time – Verification Chart

Skills	Individual Skills	Simulation/Random	Integrated into AT
Range of Motion		Range of Motion	
Strength		Strength	
Coordination/NM control		Coordination/NM control	
Functional/Sport Specific		Functional/Sport Specific	

Observer/date _____ _____ _____

Scoring Rubrics on pages 305–306

THERAPEUTIC EXERCISE – ARM AND ELBOW

Learning Over Time – Verification Chart

Skills	Individual Skills	Simulation/Random	Integrated into AT
Range of Motion		Range of Motion	
Strength		Strength	
Coordination/NM control		Coordination/NM control	
Functional/Sport Specific		Functional/Sport Specific	

Observer/date _____ _____ _____

Scoring Rubrics on pages 307–308

THERAPEUTIC EXERCISE – WRIST AND HAND

Learning Over Time – Verification Chart

Skills	Individual Skills	Simulation/Random	Integrated into AT
Range of Motion		Range of Motion	
Strength		Strength	
Coordination/NM control		Coordination/NM control	
Functional/Sport Specific		Functional/Sport Specific	

Observer/date   _____   _____   _____

Scoring Rubrics on pages 309–310

JOINT MOBILIZATION, AQUATIC THERAPY, AND PNF

Learning Over Time – Verification Chart

Skills	Individual Skills	Simulation/Random	Integrated into AT
Joint Mobilization		Joint Mobilization	
Ankle			
Knee			
Hip			
Vertebrae			
Shoulder			
Elbow			
Wrist			
Fingers & Thumb			
Aquatic Therapy		Aquatic Therapy	
Upper Body Injuries			

Lower Body Injuries			
PNF		PNF	
Upper Extremity – DI			
Upper Extremity – D2			
Lower Extremity – D1			
Lower Extremity – D2			

Observer/date _____   _____   _____

Scoring Rubrics on pages 311–313

POWER, AGILITY, SPEED, ENDURANCE

Learning Over Time – Verification Chart

Skills	Individual Skills	Simulation/Random	Integrated into AT
Lower Body		Lower Body	
Power			
Agility			
Speed			
Endurance			
Upper Body		Upper Body	
Power			
Agility			
Speed			
Power			

Observer/date _____   _____   _____

Scoring Rubrics on pages 314–315

Challenge Assignments

1. Teach an underclass student 5 rehabilitation exercises.
2. Write a synopsis of a chosen exercise. Include how to perform the exercise, muscle tissue stressed, objective of the exercise, precautions, indications and contraindications, and short- and long-term goals of the exercise.
3. Write the rehabilitation goals for a patient with whom you are working.
4. Recall an exercise you have used recently in rehabilitation. What evidence do you have that the exercise accomplishes what you want?
5. Make a table of exercises used to recondition a variety of lower body injuries. In the first column list the injuries. In the second column list the criteria you would use to determine that an exercise is appropriate/necessary for the patient. In the third column list the criteria that indicate the exercise is no longer needed for rehabilitation. Repeat this assignment for upper body injuries.
6. Explain how you would alter an athlete's lower body conditioning routine if he/she was suffering from patella femoral pain.
7. Explain how you would alter an athlete's upper body conditioning routine if he/she was suffering from shoulder instability brought on by a labrum tear.
8. Review the literature to find evidence that the exercises chosen and the prescription of sets/reps match your rehabilitation goals.

Journaling

Summarize the real-life experiences you have had with Conditioning and Rehabilitative Exercises. How have they helped your professional growth?

Date	CI/Rotation	Experience

Date	CI/Rotation	Experience

Pharmacology

A complete treatment plan may include pharmaceuticals.

Pharmaceutical Interventions

Treatment/management of injuries and illness often involves both physical and pharmaceutical interventions. A coordinated management plan allows optimal benefits to the patient. The athletic trainer may not prescribe medications; however, he/she needs to have a good working knowledge of indications, contraindications, and effects of a variety of pharmaceutical agents. The purpose of this chapter is to provide the athletic training student with the opportunity to apply his/her knowledge of pharmaceutical agents in real situations. This practice should help the AT student learn how to coordinate physical and pharmaceutical interventions to optimize the healing environment.

Background Knowledge

In order for students to maximize their professional growth in this content area they must be able to:

1. Separate drugs into appropriate classifications.
2. List the indications, contraindications, precautions, and adverse reactions of common drugs.
3. Recall typical administration techniques of common drugs and explain general advantages and disadvantages of each administration technique.
4. Explain roles and responsibilities of regulatory acts/agencies (e.g., state law, FDA, controlled substance act).
5. Define pharmacokinetic and pharmacodynamic terms (e.g., absorption, distribution, metabolism, elimination, half-life, bioequivalence, dose response, potency).
6. Delineate drug testing procedures.
7. Use a drug reference guide.
8. Recall chemical, trade, and generic names of common medications.
9. Recall proper storage factors.
10. Explain some of the procedures and main concerns with drug testing.

Goals

Write your goals that correspond to the content of this chapter.

Goal #	Goal

Discussion between the Student and ACI/CI

1. Have you ever had a patient experience an adverse reaction to a drug? What was the situation?

    _____

    _____

    _____

    _____

    _____

2. What medications do you have available for patient use? How do you store and distribute these medications?

    _____

    _____

    _____

    _____

    _____

3. What policies/laws are in place to safeguard against illicit use of medications?

    _____

    _____

    _____

    _____

    _____

4. Have you ever had an athlete fail a drug test?

    _____

    _____

    _____

    _____

5. What would you do if you suspected a co-worker or an athlete of drug abuse?

    _____

    _____

    _____

    _____

Reflection

1. Describe a situation in which a patient was taking medication. What effect did this have on his/her activity?

   _____

   _____

   _____

   _____

   _____

2. Describe a situation in which a patient had an adverse reaction to medication. Could this reaction have been predicted and/or prevented?

   _____

   _____

   _____

   _____

   _____

3. Recall a situation in which a patient had incomplete or misinformation about a pharmaceutical agent.

   _____

   _____

   _____

   _____

   _____

4. Explain a situation in which one athlete used another athlete's medication. Were there any adverse effects? What concerns do you have about this?

   _____

   _____

   _____

   _____

5. What is something that you saw that confused you?

   _____

   _____

   _____

   _____

6. What did you learn that seems to contradict what you learned from books or professors?

_____

_____

_____

_____

_____

Skills To Be Practiced and Assessed

EpiPen

Inhaler

Insulin Injection

DRUG ADMINISTRATION ASSISTANCE

Learning Over Time – Verification Chart

Skill	Individual Skills	Simulation/Random	Integrated into AT
EpiPen Administration			
Teach proper use of asthma inhaler			
Assist with insulin injection			

Observer/date   _____   _____   _____

Scoring Rubrics on pages 316–317

Challenge Assignments

1. Look up each of the drugs taken by athletes on a specific team in a pharmacology reference book (e.g., PDR) and review the indications, contraindications, recommended uses, and typical dose of each drug.
2. Critically review your school's drug testing procedures for thoroughness, fairness, and potential to detect or prevent drug use.
3. Teach an underclass student about the effects of 5 commonly used over the counter drugs.
4. Review the NCAA banned substance list. What types of substances are banned? Why?
5. Describe a situation in which an athlete was advised to take some medicine (the advice could have come from an MD, ATC, PT, parent, player, etc.). Were there any problems? Was this advice appropriate? What potential problems could arise?
6. Make a list of common drugs and list concerns you have about the drug. For example, diuretics can predispose a person to heat illness.
7. Write a scenario in which an athletic trainer would need to activate the poison control center.
8. Write a summary of the NCAA position on over-the-counter and prescription drug use.

Journaling

Summarize the real-life experiences you have had that relate to Pharmacology. How have these experiences helped your professional growth?

Date	CI/Rotation	Experience

Date	CI/Rotation	Experience

Psychosocial Intervention and Referral

The connection between mind and body is never so obvious as when one of them is under great stress.

Psychosocial Pathologies

Physically active people play a variety of games that require multiple skills. The differences between a collegiate wrestler and an elderly fitness walker may be substantial. Because these individuals are very different from each other and different from the typical population, their medical needs must be attended to by a professional with specific knowledge of their anatomy, physiology, and activity demands. While physically active people have tremendous differences they all have one similarity—they are people. All people are susceptible to psychosocial conditions such as stress and depression. The effective athletic trainer possesses the knowledge to recognize atypical behavior. Behavior may be pathological (e.g., depression leading to suicide), or it may be relatively benign yet negatively affect injury recovery (e.g., lack of motivation to rehabilitate). While the athletic trainer may not provide the primary psychosocial treatment, he/she must be able to recognize signs of psychosocial conditions, refer the person to the appropriate professional, and complement the prescribed treatment. The purpose of this chapter is to provide students with an opportunity to utilize their knowledge of psychosocial pathologies to facilitate optimal intervention and treatment.

Background Knowledge

In order for students to maximize their professional growth in this content area they must be able to:

1. Describe the role and scope of practice of psychologists, counselors, social workers, and human resources personnel.
2. Explain the role of stress, visualization, relaxation, mental preparation, and desensitizing techniques in athletic performance and injury management.
3. Explain how psychosocial factors affect pain perception and persistence.
4. Explain the grieving process.
5. Identify the signs and symptoms of addictive behavior, stress, anxiety, and substance abuse.
6. Identify the signs and symptoms of eating disorders.
7. Appropriately intervene when substance abuse is suspected.
8. Use appropriate motivational techniques during rehabilitation.

Goals

Write your goals that correspond to the content of this chapter.

Goal #	Goal

Discussion between the Student and ACI/CI

1. Have you ever had an athlete who you knew was physically ready to return to full activity but was not mentally ready to return?

   _____

   _____

   _____

   _____

   _____

2. What techniques have you used to motivate the pessimistic patient?

   _____

   _____

   _____

   _____

   _____

3. Has a cultural difference ever interfered with providing optimal patient care? If so, how?

   _____

   _____

   _____

   _____

   _____

4. Have you ever had an athlete with an eating disorder? Was the disorder ever resolved?

   _____

   _____

   _____

   _____

   _____

5. Have you had a patient who has needed psychosocial intervention in order to recover fully from an injury/illness?

   _____

   _____

   _____

   _____

   _____

6. What are some of the pre-competition or daily rituals your athletes go through?

_____
_____
_____
_____
_____

7. Have you ever had an athlete whose nervous behavior led to injury or illness?

_____
_____
_____
_____
_____

8. How do you know that someone needs psychosocial intervention beyond your scope or ability?

_____
_____
_____
_____
_____

9. What resources are available for an athlete who needs psychosocial intervention?

_____
_____
_____
_____
_____

Reflection

1. Describe a situation in which a person's psychological state influenced his/her recovery. The influence may be either positive or negative.

_____
_____
_____
_____

2. Recall a situation in which the emotional state of a coach, family member, or friend influenced the patient. What will you do in the future to make sure that others do not negatively influence your patients?

_____

_____

_____

_____

_____

3. What situations in this clinical rotation have caused you to experience stress? What have you done to deal with that stress?

_____

_____

_____

_____

_____

4. Describe a patient's psychological/emotional reaction to an injury that occurred during your clinical rotation. How do you expect the reaction to influence his/her recovery?

_____

_____

_____

_____

_____

5. Explain how your clinical instructor handles stress. Is this effective? Why or why not? Will this method work for you? Why or why not?

_____

_____

_____

_____

6. Describe a personality trait of your clinical instructor that is positive for that person but would not work for you. Explain why.

_____

_____

_____

_____

7. Choose a team or group of athletes or an individual athlete and explain how they think. What is important to them? How do they react to injuries?

_____

_____

_____

_____

_____

8. Choose one of your patients. What motivates him/her?

_____

_____

_____

_____

_____

9. What motivates your clinical instructor?

_____

_____

_____

_____

_____

10. Study your assigned team. Predict each person's reaction to a season-ending injury.

_____

_____

_____

_____

_____

11. What did you learn today that seems to contradict what you learned from books or professors?

_____

_____

_____

_____

_____

Skills To Be Practiced and Assessed

None

Challenge Assignments

1. List the signs and symptoms of eating disorders.
2. Make a list of people/agencies that you can use if psychosocial intervention is needed.
3. Choose one behavior of an athlete that interferes with success. What would you do to help him/her reduce/eliminate this behavior?
4. Develop a plan to help reduce the stress levels of your athletes.
5. Describe a situation in which a patient needed emotional support from his/her athletic trainer. In your opinion did the AT meet the patient's needs? Will you be able to provide emotional support to your future patients?
6. Describe a situation in which an athlete complained excessively or frequently to the AT. How did the AT deal with the situation? What will your strategy be for the chronic complainer?
7. Describe a situation in which an athlete did not report symptoms appropriately or early enough. How did the AT deal with the situation? What will your strategy be for dealing with athletes who hide injuries?

Journaling

Summarize the real-life Psychosocial Intervention and Referral experiences you have had. How have these experiences helped your professional growth?

Date	CI/Rotation	Experience

Date	CI/Rotation	Experience

CHAPTER 14

Nutritional Aspects of Injuries and Illnesses

Proper fuel allows for proper movement and recovery.

Nutrition

Active individuals need to follow sound nutritional practices in order to facilitate optimal performance and recovery from injury/illness. The athletic trainer needs to have a good working knowledge of nutrition in order to counsel an athlete on proper nutrition. This chapter provides the student with an opportunity to integrate his/her knowledge of nutrition into practical situations. The objective of this chapter is for students to become more comfortable and confident in their knowledge of nutrition.

Background Knowledge

In order for students to maximize their professional growth in this content area they must:

1. Explain the role of fluids, carbohydrates, protein, fat, electrolytes, vitamins, and minerals in nutrition.
2. Explain recommended daily nutritional requirements as per the USDA pyramid.
3. Explain the use of macro and micronutrients in the body.
4. List the nutritional concerns for injury and rehabilitation.

Goals

Write your goals that correspond to the content of this chapter.

Goal #	Goal

Discussion between the Student and ACI/CI

1. Have you ever had a patient whose poor nutritional habits negatively influenced injury recovery?

    _____

    _____

    _____

    _____

    _____

2. What ergogenic aids might benefit your athletes? What dangers are posed by each ergogenic aid?

    _____

    _____

    _____

    _____

    _____

3. Have you ever had an athlete who was too heavy? What did you do to modify his/her diet in order to help him/her lose weight?

    _____

    _____

    _____

    _____

    _____

4. Have you ever had an athlete who was losing weight too rapidly? What did you do to try to slow or stop the weight loss?

    _____

    _____

    _____

    _____

    _____

5. What have been some of the popular/fad diets your athletes have tried? How have these diets affected them?

    _____

    _____

    _____

    _____

    _____

6. Have you had an athlete whose poor diet resulted in illness?

    _____

    _____

    _____

    _____

Reflection

1. Reflect on the positive nutritional practices of your team members. What can you do to encourage good nutrition of your future clients/patients?

   _____

   _____

   _____

   _____

   _____

2. Reflect on the poor nutritional practices of your team members. What can you do to change their eating habits?

   _____

   _____

   _____

   _____

   _____

3. In the future what do you plan to do to ensure good nutrition of your clients?

   _____

   _____

   _____

   _____

   _____

4. What did you learn today that seems to contradict what you learned from books or professors?

   _____

   _____

   _____

   _____

   _____

Skills To Be Practiced and Assessed

None

Challenge Assignments

1. Analyze a pre-game meal of your athletes. How could it be improved?
2. Analyze a post-game meal of your athletes. How could it be improved?
3. Design a pre-game meal for your assigned athletic team.
4. Make suggestions for food to be eaten between tournament games.
5. Answer a nutrition question from one of your athletes.
6. Explain the role of iron, calcium, Vitamin A, B, C, D, E in an athlete's diet.
7. Estimate calorie intake and expenditure for one of your athletes for 1 day or 1 week.
8. Determine nutrient intake of one of your athletes for 1 day or 1 week.
9. Present a nutrition lecture to your athletes based on questions that the athletes have asked.

10. Develop a plan to recognize and treat eating disorders. Be sure to include all professionals who may need to be involved in managing patients with eating disorders.
11. Develop a weight reduction diet for one of your athletes.
12. Develop a diet to increase weight of one of your athletes.
13. Review the supplements taken by your athletes to determine the nutritional value and ergogenic benefits. Does this match the label or claims?
14. Find and summarize position papers by the NATA and other organizations that deal with nutrition, supplements, or hydration.
15. Make a list of common illnesses and injuries associated with poor nutrition.
16. Take a stand for sports drinks or water for your team. Write a paper persuading others to agree with your position.

Journaling

Summarize the real-life experiences you have had with Nutritional Aspects of Injuries and Illness. How have these experiences helped your professional growth?

Date	CI/Rotation	Experience

Date	CI/Rotation	Experience

CHAPTER 15

Health Care Administration

Proper organization allows the athletic trainer to manage the many facets of athletic training.

Administrative Practices in Health Care

Administering health care programs requires attention to detail and good communication practices. Proper administration allows for efficient health care. In order to administer health care, the AT needs to have a good working knowledge of all guidelines that affect athletic training. These guidelines come from the state government, professional organizations, and employers. This chapter is designed to provide students with the opportunity to apply their knowledge of Health Care Administration practices.

Background Knowledge

In order for students to maximize their professional growth in this content area they must:

1. Explain personnel management duties including: recruitment and selection of employees, retention of employees, development of policies and procedures manuals, administration of employment performance evaluations, and implementation of nondiscriminatory employment practices.
2. Explain the role of OSHA and other agencies/policies in prevention of communicable diseases.
3. Outline employment regulations such as the Americans with Disabilities Act (ADA), Family and Medical Leave Act (FMLA), Family Educational Rights and Privacy Act (FERPA), Fair Labor Standards Act, Equal Employment Opportunity Commission (EEOC), and Sexual Harassment.
4. Explain the role of insurance in medical care.
5. Write and evaluate a mission and vision statement.
6. Evaluate a program and personnel for effectiveness toward satisfying the employer's mission.
7. Overview the mission and organizational structure of the National Athletic Trainers' Association (NATA), Board of Certification (BOC), Commission on Accreditation of Athletic Training Education (CAATE), Journal of Athletic Training (JAT), Athletic Training Education Journal (ATEJ), and your state athletic training organization.

Goals

Write your goals that correspond to the content of this chapter.

Goal #	Goal

Discussion between the Student and ACI/CI

1. How did you decide who was going to be the team physician? What would you do differently if you were to start all over again?

_____

_____

_____

_____

_____

2. What policies should the student be aware of during the clinical rotation?

_____

_____

_____

_____

_____

3. What do you like and not like about your facilities?

_____

_____

_____

_____

_____

4. Explain how your insurance policy works.

_____

_____

_____

_____

_____

5. How do you ensure ethical treatment of all people?

_____

_____

_____

_____

_____

6. What is your primary means of communicating with physicians? coaches? parents? athletes? Is this effective?

_____

_____

_____

_____

7. What procedure do you follow to schedule an appointment with a physician?

_____

_____

_____

_____

_____

8. What advice about policy, procedures, and the administration would you give a new AT coming into your position?

_____

_____

_____

_____

_____

9. Are there any employer policies that do not make sense for AT?

_____

_____

_____

_____

_____

Reflection

1. Revisit the pre-participation physical examination form and procedure used at your clinical setting. What can you do to make it 1) more efficient and 2) more beneficial to you and the athlete regarding health information obtained?

_____

_____

_____

_____

_____

2. Could you perform the duties of your clinical instructor? If not, what do you need to do/know in order to perform his/her duties?

_____

_____

_____

_____

_____

3. Are the AT, coaches, and athletes treated fairly by each other and the administration? Would you do anything different to ensure fair treatment of people?

_____

_____

_____

_____

_____

4. Recall all the recordkeeping systems and forms with which you have worked. What are three things you want to incorporate into your recordkeeping system?

_____

_____

_____

_____

_____

5. Describe two situations that appear to be similar in pathology that were treated differently. Do you have any ideas why they were treated differently? For example, you may have witnessed two ankle injuries. The contradiction/confusion may be that one was treated with ice and the other with muscle stimulation.

_____

_____

_____

_____

_____

6. Recall three problems you have noticed at your clinical site. They can be big or little problems. How were they resolved? Or, how should they be resolved?

_____

_____

_____

_____

_____

7. Describe a problem you have noticed that stems from a written policy.

_____

_____

_____

_____

_____

8. Describe a personnel problem you have identified.

_____

_____

_____

_____

_____

9. What is the decision-making structure at your setting? Identify the people with personal authority. Identify the people with positional authority.

_____

_____

_____

_____

_____

10. If communication is a problem at your clinical site, identify the barriers to good communication.

_____

_____

_____

_____

_____

11. How do coaches, athletes, and others view your clinical instructor? Would they view you the same way if you assumed your clinical instructor's position?

_____

_____

_____

_____

12. What contribution does your clinical instructor make to the mission of his/her organization? (It is okay to ask your clinical instructor the mission of his/her organization. You should then try to determine his/her contribution.)

_____

_____

_____

_____

_____

13. Describe how you communicate with patients. Do you use humor? Are you direct? Are you sarcastic? How is your communication different with males, females? How do you communicate with those you know well and those you do not know well? How do you communicate with peers, superiors?

_____

_____

_____

_____

_____

14. Describe your ideal colleagues. Assume you are interviewing candidates to work with you. What questions would you ask to make sure there is a good fit?

_____

_____

_____

_____

_____

15. What have you learned about working with coaches? parents? medical professionals? athletic trainers?

_____

_____

_____

_____

_____

16. Describe a situation in which a patient, parent, physician, coach, AT, or administrator was disappointed, upset. What made him/her upset? What can you do to prevent this situation or a similar one in the future?

_____

_____

_____

_____

_____

17. Is this clinical setting unique in any way? How?

_____

_____

_____

_____

_____

18. Take a stance for or against a policy that affects athletic trainers. Provide your rationale for supporting or not supporting this policy.

_____

_____

_____

_____

_____

19. Describe a situation involving sensitive information (e.g., records, private communication, etc.) that was not handled very well. What lessons did you learn? What will you do when you are in a similar situation?

_____

_____

_____

_____

_____

20. What did you learn today that seems to contradict what you learned from books or professors?

_____

_____

_____

_____

_____

Challenge Assignments

1. Review the forms and recordkeeping system used in the AT facility. What modifications could you make to ensure greater efficiency and usefulness?
2. Write the initial injury/illness report on five patients.
3. Write update reports/progress notes on five patients.
4. Review a patient's file. Assign International Classification of Diseases, Ninth Revision, Clinical Modification (ICD-9-CM) and Current Procedural Terminology (CPT) codes to the evaluation and treatment performed. How could the recordkeeping system be changed to more easily affix ICD and CPT codes to patient diagnoses and treatments?
5. Write the end-of-season injury report for the team with which you are working.
6. Design a mock emergency scenario and have the ATs and AT students manage the situation.
7. Walk through the AT facility. Identify any potential hazards. Which hazards can be rectified with policy/practice, and which hazards need facility modifications?
8. Write a letter to the editor of the local paper promoting the profession of athletic training.
9. Teach underclass students about the different professionals involved with sports medicine. Include education, responsibilities, and scope of practice.
10. Redesign your clinical facility to better meet the needs of your CI and patients.
11. Review the Emergency Action Plan (EAP) for your clinical venue. Is there any situation not covered? If so, rewrite to cover all situations.
12. Order supplies for your CI.
13. Describe the dress code at your clinical setting. How would changing the dress code change the atmosphere?

Skills To Be Practiced and Assessed

Recordkeeping

RECORDKEEPING

Learning Over Time – Verification Chart

Skill	Individual skills	Simulation/Random	Integrated into AT
Injury report			
Progress/rehabilitation report			

Observer/date   _____   _____   _____

Scoring Rubrics on pages 318–319

Journaling

Summarize the real-life Health Care Administration experiences you have had. How have they helped your professional growth?

Date	CI/Rotation	Experience

Date	CI/Rotation	Experience

Professional Development Responsibilities

Professional development is a lifelong activity. It helps ensure the vitality of both the individual and the organization.

Professional Development

The knowledge and skill acquired in entry-level education allows a person to begin working in the field of athletic training. Athletic training knowledge and skill do not end with graduation or with passing the BOC certification examination. The AT has a need and a responsibility to continue learning and developing his/her skills. Without such professional development the AT would soon be using outdated information. This chapter provides an opportunity for students to build the foundation for future professional development.

Background Knowledge

In order for students to maximize their professional growth in this content area they must:

1. Compare and contrast registration, licensure, and certification.
2. List state law requirements.
3. List BOC CEU requirements.
4. Explain how the following affect the practice of athletic training: Athletic Training Educational Competencies, Standards of Practice, Code of Ethics, Role Delineation Study, CAATE, BOC, NATA, and state organizations.
5. Summarize the main ideas in the NATA position statements.
6. Summarize the main ideas in the NCAA position statements.

Goals

Write your goals that correspond to the content of this chapter.

Goal #	Goal

Discussion between the Student and ACI/CI

1. What criteria do you use when making return to play decisions?

   _____

   _____

   _____

   _____

   _____

2. What legal issues affect AT's in your state?

   _____

   _____

   _____

   _____

   _____

3. Find something in a book that contradicts what you have learned in clinical education. Discuss this difference with your CI.

   _____

   _____

   _____

   _____

   _____

4. What qualifications would the CI look for in an assistant AT?

   _____

   _____

   _____

   _____

   _____

5. What is your involvement with professional organizations? How has this impacted your practice as an AT?

   _____

   _____

   _____

   _____

   _____

6. Do you know any AT who violated state law, NATA Code of Ethics, or BOC Standards of Practice? What was the situation?

   _____

   _____

   _____

   _____

Reflection

1. What is something that you saw that confused you?

_____

_____

_____

_____

_____

2. What is one problem you see at the local level that is also a national problem/issue?

_____

_____

_____

_____

_____

3. What extraneous variables affect your clinical instructor? How does he/she deal with them?

_____

_____

_____

_____

_____

4. What motivates your clinical instructor? How does this compare to what motivates you?

_____

_____

_____

_____

_____

5. Explain the involvement of your clinical instructor in the profession of athletic training or other professions. Does this help or hinder his/her performance? How?

_____

_____

_____

_____

_____

6. We all function best when our environment is ideal for us. What questions will you ask during your job interview to determine if the environment is right for you?

_____

_____

_____

_____

_____

7. What are your professional goals? What is your plan to achieve your goals? In your plan begin by stating what you can do as a student.

_____

_____

_____

_____

_____

8. What challenges do you perceive for yourself if you were to have your clinical instructor's job tomorrow? What would you need to do to prepare for the patient load? What would you need to do to prepare to work with your new coworkers? What areas of expertise would you need to possess?

_____

_____

_____

_____

_____

9. Explain the single most challenging aspect of your current clinical setting. Why is it so challenging?

_____

_____

_____

_____

_____

10. Fear of the unknown is one of the greatest fears in life. To help future students reduce their level of anxiety when they come to this clinical setting, what advice do you have for them?

_____

_____

_____

_____

_____

11. What did you learn today that seems to contradict what you learned from books or professors?

_____

_____

_____

_____

_____

Skills To Be Assessed

None

Challenge Assignments

1. Summarize the position statements of the NATA.
2. Describe the scope of practice of all health care professionals with whom you have come in contact.
3. Find 10 web sites of organizations that assist the athletic trainer with continuing education.
4. Design an injury prevention program for the athletes with whom you work.
5. Find a position announcement on the NATA Career Center and write a resume and letter of application for this position.
6. The following are dimensions of professional competence. Rate yourself in each of the following areas with 1 = very weak to 5 = very strong. Then explain your plan to ensure that you continue with your strengths and make adjustment to areas in which you are weak.
   Communication skills
   Knowledge
   Ability to handle stress
   Technical skills
   Clinical reasoning
   Patient interaction
   Problem solving
   Attention to detail
   Patient care
   Curiosity
   Self-awareness
   Ability to identify and correct errors
7. Attend a professional conference. While at the conference:
   a. Introduce yourself to an AT leader (you can define leader). Ask his/her advice on obtaining a job, advanced education, or any issue that is pertinent to AT.
   b. Critically review a presentation for use of evidence to support the presenter's claims.
8. Summarize what you need to do to a) become certified, b) maintain certification, c) become licensed/certified in your state, and d) maintain state credentialing.
9. Ask your CI or faculty member to conduct a mock interview.
10. Join the NATA if you are not already a member.
11. Email the president of your state athletic training organization and ask how you can get involved with the state organization—follow through.

Journaling

Summarize the real-life Professional Development experiences you have had. How have they helped your professional growth?

Date	CI/Rotation	Experience

Date	CI/Rotation	Experience

SECTION 3

Reference Material

CHAPTER 17

Muscles – Attachments, Actions, Innervation

Students should be able to list the muscles that act on each joint. They should also be able to list the attachment points and nerve innervations of each muscle. With this information the informed student will be able to assess the strength of each muscle. He/she will also be able to develop reconditioning exercises that strengthen each muscle.

INTRINSIC FOOT

Muscle	Proximal Attachment	Distal Attachment	Action	Innervation
Flexor Digitorum Brevis	plantar surface of calcaneus	medial and lateral surfaces of middle 2nd, 3rd, 4th, 5th phalanges	MP and PIP flexion of 2nd, 3rd, 4th, 5th phalanges	Medial Plantar Nerve
Abductor Digiti Minimi	plantar surface of calcaneus	lateral surface of 5th proximal phalanx	abduction of 5th phalange at MP	Lateral Plantar Nerve
Flexor Hallucis Brevis	cuboid and lateral cuneiform	medial surface 1st proximal phalanx; lateral surface 1st proximal phalanx	flexion of 1st phalange at MP	Medial Plantar Nerve
Abductor Hallucis	plantar surface of calcaneus, flexor retinaculum, plantar aponeurosis	medial surface base of 1st proximal phalanx	abduction 1st phalanx, flexion 1st MP	Medial Plantar Nerve
Flexor Digiti Minimi Brevis	base of 5th metatarsal	lateral surface 5th proximal phalanx	flexion of MP of 5th phalange	Lateral Plantar Nerve

(continues)

INTRINSIC FOOT (*continued*)

Muscle	Proximal Attachment	Distal Attachment	Action	Innervation
Quadratus Plantae	medial surface of calcaneus; lateral inferior surface of calcaneus	lateral border of the flexor digitorum longus tendon	flexion of DIP of 2nd, 3rd, 4th, 5th, phalanges	Lateral Plantar Nerve
Lumbricles	flexor digitorum longus tendons	dorsal surface 2nd, 3rd, 4th, 5th proximal phalanges	flexion of MP of 2nd, 3rd, 4th, 5th, phalanges	1st Lumbricles Medial Plantar Nerve
				2nd–4th Lumbricles Lateral Plantar Nerve
Adductor Hallucis	2nd, 3rd, 4th, 5th metatarsals	lateral surface base of 1st proximal phalanx	adduction 1st phalange at MP	Lateral Plantar Nerve
Plantar Interossei	medial surfaces of 3rd, 4th and 5th metatarsals	medial surface 3rd, 4th, 5th proximal phalanges	flexion 3rd, 4th, 5th phalanges at MP; MP adduction	Lateral Plantar Nerve
Dorsal Interossei	metatarsals	medial surface 2nd proximal phalanx; lateral surface 2nd, 3rd, 4th proximal phalanges	flexion 3rd, 4th, 5th phalanges at MP; MP abduction	Lateral Plantar Nerve
Extensor Digitorum Brevis	dorsal surface calcaneus	proximal 1st phalanx; lateral border extensor digitorum longus tendon 2nd, 3rd, 4th phalanges	extension of first 4 toes	Deep Peroneal Nerve

FOOT AND ANKLE

Muscle	Proximal Attachment	Distal Attachment	Action	Innervation
Plantaris	lateral femoral epicondyle	calcaneus along medial side of achilles tendon	plantar flexion of ankle; knee flexion	Tibial Nerve
Gastrocnemius	posterior surface of medial and lateral femoral condyles	posterior surface of the calcaneus via the achilles tendon	plantar flexion of ankle; knee flexion	Tibial Nerve
Soleus	posterior surface of the proximal fibula and posterior surface of the proximal 2/3 of the tibia	posterior surface of the calcaneus via the achilles tendon	plantar flexion of the ankle	Tibial Nerve
Tibialis Posterior	posterior interosseus membrane and adjacent tibia and fibula	plantar surfaces of navicular, cuneiform, and base of 2nd, 3rd, 4th, 5th metatarsals	inverson of ankle; plantar flexion of ankle	Tibial Nerve
Flexor Digitorus Longus	middle 1/3 posterior surface of tibia	plantar surface of base of the 2nd, 3rd, 4th , 5th distal phalanges	flexion of 4 toes; plantar flexion of ankle	Tibial Nerve
Flexor Hallucis Longus	middle 2/3 posterior surface of fibula	plantar surface of base of the distal phalanx of great toe	flexion of great toe; plantar flexion of ankle	Tibial Nerve
Peroneus Longus	proximal 2/3 of lateral surface of the fibula	plantar surface of medial (1st) cuneiform and 1st metatarsal	eversion of ankle; plantar flexion of ankle	Superficial Peroneal Nerve
Peroneus Brevis	distal 1/3 of lateral surface of fibula	tuberosity of the 5th metatarsal	eversion of ankle; plantar flexion of ankle	Superficial Peroneal Nerve
Peroneus Tertius	distal 1/3 of anterior surface of fibula	base of 5th metatarsal	eversion of ankle; dorsiflexion of ankle	Deep Peroneal Nerve
Extensor Digitorum Longus	proximal 2/3 of anterior surface of the fibula	dorsal surface of distal phalanges of 2nd, 3rd, 4th, 5th toes	toe extension; dorsiflexion of ankle	Deep Peroneal Nerve
Extensor Hallucis Longus	middle 2/3 of medial surface of the fibula	dorsal surface of the distal phalanx of great toe	great toe extension; dorsiflexion of ankle	Deep Peroneal Nerve
Tibialis Anterior	proximal 2/3 of lateral surface of the tibia	medial (1st) cuneiform and base of 1st metatarsal	dorsiflexion of ankle; inversion of ankle	Deep Peroneal Nerve

KNEE

Muscle	Proximal Attachment	Distal Attachment	Action	Innervation
Semitendinosus	ischial tuberosity	pes anserine	extension of hip; flexion of knee; medial rotation of tibia	Tibial Nerve
Semimembranosus	ischial tuberosity	posterior medial tibial condyle	extension of hip; flexion of knee; medial rotation of tibia	Tibial Nerve
Biceps Femoris	ischial tuberosity and linea aspera	head of the fibula	extension of hip; flexion of knee; lateral rotation of tibia	Tibial Nerve – Long head Peroneal Nerve – Short head
Popliteus	posterior surface of lateral condyle of femur	posterior medial surface of tibia	medial rotation of tibia; flexion of knee	Tibal Nerve
Rectus Femoris	AIIS	tibial tuberosity via patella tendon	flexion of hip; extension of knee	Femoral Nerve
Vastus Lateralis	linea aspera and lateral femur	tibial tuberosity via patella tendon	extension of knee	Femoral Nerve
Vastus Intermedius	anterior surface of femur	tibial tuberosity via patella tendon	extension of knee	Femoral Nerve
Vastus Medialis	linea aspera and medial femur	tibial tuberosity via patella tendon	extension of knee	Femoral Nerve

HIP

Muscle	Proximal Attachment	Distal Attachment	Action	Innervation
Sartorius	ASIS	pes anserine	flexion, adduction, lateral rotation of the hip; flexion of knee; medial rotation of tibia	Femoral Nerve
Iliacus	inner surface of ilium	lesser trochanter of femur	flexion of hip; external rotation of femur	Lumbar and Femoral Nerve
Psoas Major	transverse processes, vertebral bodies and intervertebral discs of T12–L5	lesser trochanter of femur	flexion of hip; external rotation of femur	Lumbar and Femoral Nerve
Pectineus	pubis	medial superior femur near lesser trochanter	flexion of hip; adduction of hip; internal rotation of hip	Femoral Nerve
Adductor Brevis	pubis	proximal 1/2 of linea aspera	adduction of hip	Obturator Nerve

Muscle	Proximal Attachment	Distal Attachment	Action	Innervation
Adductor Longus	pubis	middle 1/3 of linea aspera	adduction of hip	Obturator Nerve
Adductor Magnus	pubic ramus, ischial ramus	entire length of linea aspera, adductor tubercle	adduction of hip; assists with hip extension when in flexed position	Obturator Nerve and Tibial Nerve
Gracilis	pubis	pes anserine of tibia	adduction of hip; flexion of knee; internal rotation of hip	Obturator Nerve
Semitendinosus	ischial tuberosity	pes anserine of tibia	flexion of knee; extension of hip; internal rotation of hip; internal rotation of tibia	Tibial Nerve
Semimembranosus	ischial tuberosity	posterior medial tibial condyle	flexion of knee; extension of hip; internal rotation of hip; internal rotation of tibia	Tibial Nerve
Biceps Femoris	long head: ischial tuberosity; short head: distal ½ of linea aspera and lateral condylar ridge	head of the fibula	flexion of knee; extension of hip; external rotation of hip; external rotation of tibia	Tibial Nerve
Gluteus Medius	lateral surface of ilium	greater trochanter of femur	abduction of hip	Superior Gluteal Nerve
Gluteus Minimus	lateral surface of ilium	greater trochanter of femur	abduction of hip	Superior Gluteal Nerve
Gluteus Maximus	iliac crest; sacrum; coccyx; lumbar fascia	gluteal tuberosity; iliotibial band	extension of hip; external rotation of hip	Inferior Gluteal Nerve
Deep Six Rotators** Piriformis, gemellus superior, gemellus inferior, obturator extgernus, obturator internus, quadratus femoris	anterior sacrum, ischium, obturator foramen	greater trochanter	external rotation of the hip	Sacral and Obturator Nerves
Tensor Fascia Lata	anterior iliac crest	iliotibial tract to the Gerdy's tubercle	abduction of the hip; flexion of the hip; internal rotation of the hip	Superior Gluteal Nerve

** The Deep Six Rotators are grouped together because they cannot be distinguished with assessment and are treated as a group during rehabilitation.

SCAPULA

Muscle	Proximal Attachment	Distal Attachment	Action	Innervation
Upper Trapezius	base of the skull, cervical spinous processes	posterior aspect of distal 1/3 of clavicle	elevation of shoulder; upward rotation	Spinal Accessory Nerve
Middle Trapezius	spinous processes of upper thoracic vertebrae	acromion process; spine of the scapula	elevation of shoulder; adduction of scapula; retraction of scapula	Spinal Accessory Nerve
Lower Trapezius	spinous processes lower thoracic vertebrae	spine of the scapula	depression of shoulder; downward rotation	Spinal Accessory Nerve
Rhomboids Major/ Minor	spinous processes of T1–T5	vertebral border of scapula	retraction; elevation	Dorsal Scapula Nerve
Serratus Anterior	ribs	vertebral border of scapula	protraction; upward rotation	Long Thoracic Nerve
Pectoralis Minor	ribs 3–5	coracoid process of scapula	protraction; depression; downward rotation	Medial pectoral nerve
Levator Scapulae	transverse processes of cervical vertebrae	superior angle of scapula	elevation	Dorsal Scapula Nerve

GLENOHUMERAL JOINT

Muscle	Proximal Attachment	Distal Attachment	Action	Innervation
Latissimus Dorsi	ilium; lumbar and thoracic spinous processes	medial intertubercle groove	extension, internal rotation, adduction of humerus	Thoracodorsal Nerve
Teres Major	inferior angle and lateral border of scapula	medial intertubercle groove	extension, internal rotation, adduction of humerus	Lower Subscapular Nerve
Teres Minor	lateral border of scapula	greater tubercle	external rotation; horizontal abduction	Axillary Nerve
Infraspinatus	infraspinous fossa	greater tubercle	external rotation; horizontal abduction	Suprascapula Nerve
Supraspinatus	suprascapular fossa	greater tubercle	setting of head in glenoid fossa; abduction	Suprascapula Nerve
Subscapularis	subscapular fossa	lesser tubercle	internal rotation	Subscapula Nerve
Pectoralis Major	clavicle, ribs, sternum	intertubercle groove	internal rotation; horizontal adduction; adduction	Pectoral Nerve

Muscle	Proximal Attachment	Distal Attachment	Action	Innervation
Biceps Brachii	supraglenoid tubercle and coracoid process	radial tuberosity	shoulder flexion; elbow flexion; supination	Musculocutaneous
Coracobrachialis	coracoid process	medial border of humerus	adduction; horizontal adduction	Musculocutaneous
Deltoid (A, M, P)	clavicle, acromion process, spine of scapula	deltoid tuberosity	abduction; horizontal abduction; horizontal adduction	Axillary Nerve

ELBOW

Muscle	Proximal Attachment	Distal Attachment	Action	Innervation
Biceps Brachii	supraglenoid tubercle and coracoid process	radial tuberosity	shoulder flexion; elbow flexion; supination	Musculocutaneous Nerve
Brachialis	distal half anterior humerus	coronoid process of ulna	flexion of elbow	Musculocutaneous Nerve
Brachioradialis	lateral epicondyle of humerus	styloid process of radius	flexion of elbow; assist in pronation if in supinated position; assist in supination if in pronated position	Radial Nerve
Triceps	infraglenoid tubercle; proximal posterior surface of humerus; distal 2/3 posterior surface of humerus	olecranon process of ulna	elbow extension; shoulder extension; horizontal abduction	Radial Nerve
Anconeus	lateral epicondyle of humerus	olecranon process of ulna	extension of elbow	Radial Nerve
Supinator	lateral epicondyle of humerus	proximal lateral radius	supination	Radial Nerve
Pronator Teres	medial epicondyle and medial proximal humerus	middle 1/3 of lateral radius	pronation	Median Nerve
Pronator Quadratus	distal 1/3 of anterior ulna	distal 1/3 of anterior radius	pronation	Median Nerve

WRIST

Muscle	Proximal Attachment	Distal Attachment	Action	Innervation
Palmaris Longus	medial epicondyle of humerus	palmar aponeurosis	flexion of wrist	Median Nerve
Flexor Carpi Radialis	medial epicondyle of humerus	base of 2nd and 3rd metacarpal on palmar surface	wrist flexion; radial deviation	Median Nerve
Flexor Carpi Ulnaris	medial epicondyle of humerus	base of 5th metacarpal of palmar surface	wrist flexion; ulnar deviation	Ulnar Nerve
Extensor Carpi Radialis Longus	lateral epicondyle and lateral supracondylar ridge of humerus	base of 2nd metacarpal on dorsal surface	wrist extension; radial deviation	Radial Nerve
Extensor Carpi Radialis Brevis	lateral epicondyle of humerus	base of 3rd metacarpal on dorsal surface	wrist extension; radial deviation	Radial Nerve
Extensor Carpi Ulnaris	lateral epicondyle of humerus	base of 5th metacarpal on dorsal surface	wrist extension; radial deviation	Radial Nerve
Flexor Digitorum Superficialis	medial epicondyle of humerus	middle phalanges palmar surface, both sides	flexion of fingers at MP and PIP joints; wrist flexion	Median Nerve
Flexor Digitorum Profundus	proximal 1/2 anterior and medial ulna	base of distal phalanges on four fingers	flexion of fingers at DIP, PIP and MP joints; wrist flexion	Median Nerve
Flexor Pollicis Longus	middle anterior surface of radius and anterior medial border of ulna	base of distal phalanx of thumb on palmar surface	flexion of thumb at MP joint and IP	Median Nerve

THUMB AND FINGERS

Muscle	Proximal Attachment	Distal Attachment	Action	Innervation
Extensor Digitorum	lateral epicondyle of humerus	middle and distal phalanges of 4 fingers	extension of DIP joint; extension of MP; extension of wrist	Radial Nerve
Extensor Digiti Minimi	lateral epicondyle of humerus	base of middle and distal phalanxes of little finger	extension of little finger at MP	Radial Nerve
Abductor Pollicis Longus	posterior middle radius and ulna	dorsal surface of thumb metacarpal	abduction of thumb and MP; Wrist radial deviation	Radial Nerve
Extensor Pollicis Longus	posterior surface of distal 1/2 of ulna	distal phalanx of thumb on dorsal surface	extends the thumb at DP and MP	Radial Nerve
Extensor Pollicis Brevis	posterior surface of distal 1/2 of ulna	proximal phalanx of thumb on dorsal surface	extends the thumb at MP	Radial Nerve
Extensor Indicis	distal 1/2 of the posterior ulna	base of middle and distal phalanxes of index finger	extension of index finger MP	Radial Nerve
Flexor Digitorum Superficialis	medial epicondyle of humerus	sides of the middle phalanges of 4 fingers	finger flexion at PIP and MP	Median Nerve
Flexor Digitorum Profundus	proximal 3/4 of anterior medial ulna	base of distal phalanges of 4 fingers	finger flexion at DIP, PIP, and MP	Median Nerve – 2nd and 3rd fingers; Ulnar Nerve 4th and 4th fingers
Flexor Pollicis Longus	anterior middle 1/2 radius and anterior medial border of ulna	distal phalanx of thumb on palmar surface	flexion of thumb at IP and MP	Median Nerve
Opponens Pollicis	transverse carpal ligament and trapezium	lateral border of thumb metacarpal	opposition of the thumb	Median Nerve
Abductor Pollicis Brevis	transverse carpal ligament; trapezium, scaphoid	base of proximal thumb phalanx	abduction of thumb	Median Nerve
Flexor Pollicis Brevis	superficial head: transverse carpal ligament; trapezium; deep head: thumb metacarpal	base of proximal thumb phalanx	flexion and abduction at the CM; Flexion of MP	Superficial Head: Median Nerve; Deep Head: Ulnar Nerve
Adductor Pollicis	transverse head: anterior shaft of long metacarpal; oblique head: base of index and long metacarpals, capitate, and trapezoid	base of proximal thumb phalanx	adduction of CM; flexion of MP	Ulnar Nerve

(continues)

THUMB AND FINGERS (*continued*)

Muscle	Proximal Attachment	Distal Attachment	Action	Innervation
Lumbricles	flexor digitorum profundus tendon	extensor expansions on radial side of proximal phalanges of fingers	Flexion of MP	Median Nerve Lumbricles to 2nd & 3rd finger; Ulnar Nerve Lumbricles to 4th and 5th fingers
Abductor Digiti Minimi	pisiform and flexor carpi ulnaris tendon	base of 5th proximal phalanx on ulnar side	abduction of MP of little finger	Ulnar Nerve
Palmar Interossei	shaft of index, ring, and little metacarpals	base of index, ring, and little proximal phalanges	adduction of MP	Ulnar Nerve
Dorsal Interossei	shaft of metacarpals	base of index, long, ring proximal phalanges	flexion and abduction of MP	Ulnar Nerve

There are 2 naming systems for the metacarpals and phalanges. One system uses numbers 1–5 to correspond with the digits of the thumb to the little finger. For example, the metacarpal at the thumb is the 1st metacarpal. The other naming system uses Thumb, Index, Long, Ring, and Little as the names of the metacarpals. In this naming system the first metacarpal is the thumb metacarpal. The 4th metacarpal is the ring metacarpal. Either system may be used by the professionals with whom the athletic trainer works. Students should know both systems.

BACK AND NECK

Muscle	Proximal Attachment	Distal Attachment	Action	Innervation
Sternocleidomastoid	manubrium of sternum and medial clavicle	mastoid process	bilateral contraction – flexion of head and neck	Spinal Accessory Nerve
			unilateral contraction – lateral flexion to ipsilateral side; rotation to contralateral side	
Scalenes A, M, P	transverse processes C2–C7	1st and 2nd ribs	elevation of ribs; lateral flexion of neck; contralateral rotation of neck	Ventral rami of C3–C8
Levator Scapulae	transverse processes of C2–C4	superior angle of scapula	elevation of scapula	Dorsal Scapular Nerve
Splenius Cervicis	spinous process thoracic vertebrae 3–6	transverse processes C1–C3	bilateral contraction – extension of spine	Cervical Nerves
			unilateral contraction – lateral flexion to ipsilateral side	
Splenius Capitis	ligamentum nuchae; spinous processes C7–T4	mastoid process and occipital bone	bilateral contraction – extension of head	Cervical Nerves
			unilateral contraction – lateral flexion to ipsilateral side	
Iliocostalis Lumborum, Thoracis, Cervicis	thoracolumbar aponeurosis from sacrum to ribs	ribs and cervical transverse processes	bilateral contraction – extension of spine	Spinal Nerves
			unilateral contraction – lateral flexion to ipsilateral side	
Longisimus Thoracis, Cervicis, Capitus	lumbar and thoracic transverse processes	thoracic and cervical transverse processes	bilateral contraction – extension of spine	Spinal Nerves
			unilateral contraction – lateral flexion to ipsilateral side	
Spinalis – Thoracis, Cervicis, Capitus	thoracic and cervical spinous processes; ligamentum nuchae	thoracic and cervical spinous processes; occipital bone	bilateral contraction – extension of spine and head	Spinal Nerves
			unilateral contraction – lateral flexion to ipsilateral side	
Quadratus Lumborum	iliac crest	transverse processes of lumbar vertebrae and 12th rib	lateral flexion to ipsilateral side	T12–L1 Nerve roots

ABDOMEN

Muscle	Proximal Attachment	Distal Attachment	Action	Innervation
Rectus Abdominus	5th–7th ribs, xiphoid process	pubis	bilateral contraction – trunk flexion; unilateral contraction – flexion to ipsilateral side	Intercostal Nerves
External Abdominal Obliques	lower ribs	iliac crest, inguinal ligament, pubis, abdominal fascia	bilateral contraction – trunk flexion; unilateral contraction – rotation to contralateral side	Intercostal Nerves
Internal Abdominal Obliques	lower ribs and linea alba	inguinal ligament, iliac crest, lumbar fascia	bilateral contraction – trunk flexion; unilateral contraction – rotation to ipsilateral side	Intercostal Nerves
Transversus Abdominus	inguinal ligament, iliac crest, lumbar fascia, lower ribs	pubis, abdominal aponeurosis, linea alba	forced expiration	Intercostal Nerves

Palpable Structures

Students should be able to palpate the following structures or be able to palpate the location of these structures. Pain typically originates from the injured tissue. Discerning the origin of the pain will greatly assist the identification of the pathology.

FOOT/ANKLE

Bones	Soft Tissue
Medial and lateral malleolae	Deltoid ligament
Tibia	Anterior talofibular ligament
Tibiofibular Joint	Calcaneofibular ligament
Calcaneus	Extensor Tendons – Tibialis Anterior
Sustentaculum Tali	Extensor Hallucis Longus, Extensor
Medial Calcaneal Tuberosity	Digitorum Longus
Dome of the talus	Extensor Digitorum Brevis Muscle
Navicular	Plantar Fascia
Navicular tubercle	Achilles Tendon
Medial Cuneiform	Flexor Tendon Group – Tibialis
Intermediate Cuneiform	Posterior, Flexor Hallicus Longus, Flexor Digitorum
Lateral Cuneiform	Longus
Cuboid	Peroneus Longus Tendon
Base, Shaft, Head	Peroneus Brevis Tendon
Metatarsal 1–5	Interosseus space
Styloid process	
MP Joints	
Sesmoid bones	

LOWER LEG

Bones	Soft Tissue
Shaft of Tibia	Tibialis Anterior
Medial Border of the Tibia	Peroneus Longus and Brevis
Tibial Tuberosity	Peroneal tendons
Medial Tibial Plateau	Gastrocnemius
Lateral Tibial Plateau	Soleus
Pes Anserine	Achilles tendon
Gerdy's Tubercle	
Tibiofibular Joint	
Head of the Fibula	
Shaft of Fibula	

KNEE

Bones	Soft Tissue
Patella	Patella Tendon
Infrapatellar surface	Medial joint line (Meniscus)
Femoral articular surface	Lateral joint line (Meniscus)
Lateral condyle of the femur	Lateral Collateral Ligament
Medial condyle of the femur	Medial Collateral Ligament
Medial epicondyle	Popliteal space
Lateral epicondyle	Biceps Femoris Tendon
	Semimembranosus Tendon
	Semitendinosus Tendon

THIGH/HIP

Bones	Soft Tissue
Greater Trochanter	Vastus Medialis Oblique
Ischial Tuberosity	Vastus Medialis
Iliac crest	Rectus Femoris
ASIS	Vastus Lateralis
PSIS	Semitendinosus
SI joint	Semimembranosus
	Biceps Femoris
	Adductor group
	Tensor Fascia Lata
	Gluteus Maximus

BACK/NECK

Bones	Soft Tissue
Spinous Processes	Erector Spinae muscles
Ribs	Latissimus Dorsi
	Rhomboids
	Upper Trap
	Middle Trap
	Lower Trap
	Serratus Anterior

SHOULDER

Bones	Soft Tissue
Clavicle	Pectoralis Major
Sternal end	Deltoid
Body	Biceps tendon
Acromial end	Supraspinatus attachment
Coracoid process	Infraspinatus
Acromioclavicular Joint	Teres Minor
Acromion process	Triceps tendon
Spine of the scapula	Subscapularis tendon

(continues)

SHOULDER (*continued*)

Bones	Soft Tissue
Superior angle of the scapula	
Vertebral border	
Inferior angle of the scapula	
Greater Tubercle	
Lesser Tubercle	

ARM/ELBOW

Bones	Soft Tissue
Posterior Humeral Head	Triceps
Bicipital Groove	Biceps
Medial Epicondyle	Distal Triceps tendon
Lateral Epicondyle	Long Head of Biceps
Olecranon Process	Distal Biceps tendon
Ulnar Groove	Wrist flexor muscle attachment
Radial Head	Wrist extensor muscle attachment
Ulna	Wrist extensor tendons
Ulnar Tuberosity	

WRIST/HAND

Bones	Soft Tissue
Head of ulna	Extensor Pollicus Longus
Distal radius	Abductor Pollicus Longus
Radial styloid process	Anatomic snuff box
Lister's tubercle	Extensor tendons
Navicular	Thenar eminence
Lunate	Hypothenar eminence
Triquetrum	Volar plate
Hamate	Collateral ligaments
Hook of hamate	Palmaris Longus
Pisiform	

Bones	Soft Tissue
Lunate	
Capitate	
Trapezium	
Trapezoid	
Thumb metacarpal	
Index metacarpal	
Long metacarpal	
Ring metacarpal	
Little metacarpal	
Phalanges	
MP joints	

HEAD

Bones
Frontal
Parietal
Occipital
Temporal
Maxilla
Mandible
Temporomandibular Joint
Nasal

Nerves

A student who understands the anatomy of the peripheral nervous system will have a very good grasp of the entire musculoskeletal anatomy.

   You should be able to:

1. Follow the path of the nerve from its origin to its terminal end.
2. Identify the muscles innervated by each motor nerve.
3. Identify the area of sensation for each sensory nerve.
4. Cite the function of each cranial nerve.
5. Cite the nerve roots that contribute to each nerve.
6. Draw the brachial, cervical, lumbar, and sacral plexus.
7. Identify each myotome and dermatome.
8. Assess the strength of the muscles that correspond to each motor nerve.
9. Test the common deep tendon reflexes (C5, C6, C7, L4, S1).

Cranial nerves

I	Olfactory	VII	Facial
II	Optic	VIII	Vestibulocochlear
III	Oculomotor	IX	Glosopharyngeal
IV	Trochlear	X	Vagus
V	Abducens	XI	Accessory
VI	Trigeminal	XII	Hypoglossal

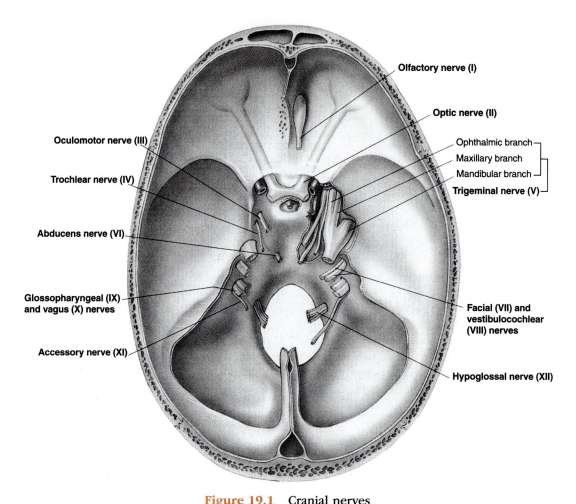

Figure 19.1 Cranial nerves

PERIPHERAL NERVES

Upper Body	Lower Body
Scapular	Superior Gluteal
Long Thoracic	Inferior Gluteal
Suprascapular	Obturator
Subclavian	Femoral
Upper Subscapular	Tibial
Lower Subscapular	Superficial Peroneal
Thoracodorsal	Deep Peroneal
Pectoral	Medial Plantar
Axillary	Lateral Plantar
Musculocutaneus	
Radial	
Median	
Ulnar	

Deep Tendon Reflex

C5 – Biceps
C6 – Brachioradialis
C7 – Triceps
L4 – Patellar Tendon
S1 – Achilles Tendon

Assessment scale

0: absent

1: trace

2: normal

3: slightly hyperactive

4: hyperactive with clonus (i.e., repetitive vibratory movements)

5: sustained clonus

SENSORY LEVELS

Hearing, equilibrium
Taste
Pharynx, esophagus
Larynx, trachea
Occipital region (C1, 2)
Neck region (C2, 3, 4)
Shoulder (C4, 5)
Axillary (C5, 6)
Radial (C6, 7, 8)
Median (C6, 7, 8)
Ulnar (C8, T1)

Arm

Spinous Processes
Spinal Nerves
First Rib

Thorax — Spine of Scapula (T3)

Epigastrium — Inferior Angle of Scapula (T7)

Abdomen

Umbilicus (T10)

Gluteal Region (T12, L1)
Inguinal region (L1, 2)

Femoral Region (L1, 2, 3) — Antrior Median Lateral Posterior

Crural Region (L4, 5) — Median Lateral

Scrotum, Penis
Labia
Perineum (S1, 2)
Bladder (S3, 4)
Rectum (S4, 5)
Anus (S5, Co1)

Filum Terminate

Medulla Oblongata

Cervical Plexus
Brachial Plexus
Intercostal and Thoracic Muscles
Abdominal Muscles
Lumbar Muscles
Lumbar Plexus
Sacral Plexus
Sacrococcygeal Plexus

MOTOR LEVELS

Facial Muscles VII
Pharyngeal, palatine muscles X
Laryngeal muscles XI
Tongue muscles XII
Esophagus X
Sternocleidomastoid XI (C1, 2, 3)
Neck muscles (C1, 2, 3)
Trapezius (C3, 4)
Rhomboids (C4, 5)
Diaphragm (C3, 4, 5)
Supra-, infraspinatus (C4, 5, 6)
Deltoid, brachioradialis, and biceps (C5, 6)
Serratus anterior (C5, 6, 7)
Pectoralis major (C5, 6, 7, 8)
Teres minor (C4, 5)
Pronators (C6, 7, 8, T1)
Triceps (C6, 7, 8)
Long extensors of carpi and digits (C6, 7, 8)
Latissimus dorsi, teres major (C5, 6, 7, 8)
Long flexors (C7, 8, T1)
Thumb extensors (C7, 8)
Interossei, lumbricales, thenar, hypothenar (C8, T1)
Iliopsoas (L1, 2, 3)
Sartorius (L2, 3)
Quadriceps femoris (L2, 3, 4)
Gluteal muscles (L4, 5, S1)
Tensor fasciae latae (L4, 5)
Adductors of femur (L2, 3, 4)
Abductors of femur (L4, 5, S1)
Tibialis anterior (L5)
Gastrocnemius, soleus (L5, S1, 2)
Biceps, semitendinosus, semimembranosus (L4, 5, S1)
Obturator, piriformis, quadratus femoris (L4, 5, S1)
Flexors of the foot, extensors of toes (L5, S1)
Peronei (L5, S1)
Flexors of toes (L5, S1, 2)
Interossei (S1, 2)
Perineal muscles (S3, 4)
Vesicular muscles (S4, 5)
Rectal muscles (S4, 5, Co1)

Arm · Forearm · Hand

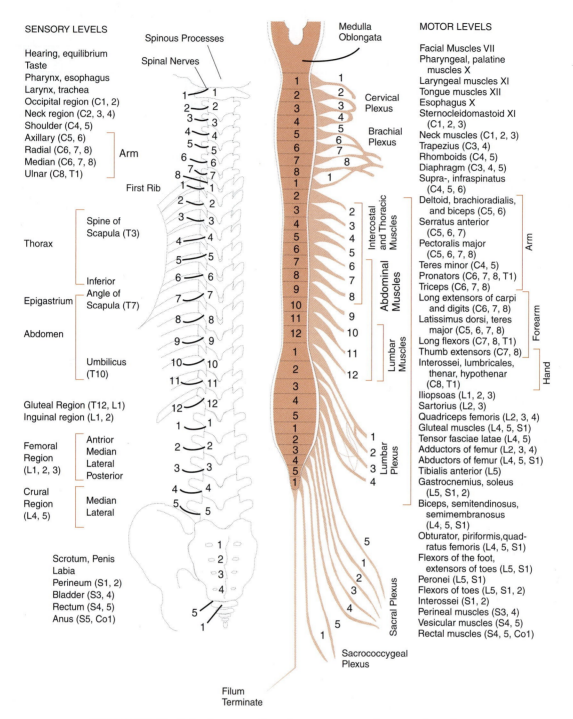

Figure 19.2   Spinal nerves showing sensory and motor functions

Assessment Tests

Athletic trainers must be able to perform and interpret many assessment tests. Complete knowledge requires a professional to be able to explain the mechanics of the test, the indications of a positive test, the pathologies that might produce a false positive test, and the limitations of each test. To have complete working knowledge of assessment tests athletic trainers should also know the approximate validity and reliability of each test.

Shoulder

Anterior drawer

Posterior drawer

Relocation test

Apprehension test

Clunk test

Sulcus sign

Speeds test

Drop-arm test

Empty can test

Hawkins-Kennedy test

Neer

Yergason

Ludington's test

Adson's maneuver

Allen test

Military brace test

Other

Elbow

Valgus

Varus

Tinel sign

Other

Neck

Nerve root compression

Spurling's test

Tinel sign

Valsalva

Other

Wrist

Finkelstein test
Valgus
Varus
Glide
Phalen's
Reverse Phalen's
Tinel sign
Other

Back

Straight-leg raise
Well-leg raise
Babinski
Kernig
Brudzinski
Hoover
Valsava
Thomas Test
Beevor's sign
Spring Test
Deep Tendon Reflex
Straight-Leg Test
Well-Leg Raise Test
Other

Hip/Pelvis

FABER (Patrick)
Pelvic compression
Pelvic distraction
Trendelenburg test
Thomas test
Ober test
Noble test
Pelvic Rock
Gaenslen's Test
Long Sit
Other

Knee

Valgus
Varus
Lachman's
Anterior drawer
Posterior drawer
Pivot shift
Q Angle Assessment
Tinel's sign
Other

Lower Leg

Homan's sign
Tib Fib Translation
Squeeze Test
Other

Ankle/Foot

Tib/Fib compression
Tap test
Anterior drawer
Posterior drawer
Inversion stress
Eversion stress
Kleiger test
Thompson test
Tinel
Navicular Drop
Morton's Neuroma (squeeze) test
Other

CHAPTER 21

Concussion Symptoms

Concussions (mild traumatic brain injury) are very common in contact sports. These injuries present a particular challenge to the Athletic Trainer because there are very few objective signs upon which to make a diagnosis. The hidden effects of the concussion may be subtle but nonetheless very dangerous. It is paramount that the Athletic Trainer has a solid working knowledge of the signs and symptoms of concussions.

Signs and Symptoms

Checklist as presented in the 2004 NATA Position Statement:

Blurred Vision	Nausea
Dizziness	Nervousness
Drowsiness	Personality change
Excess Sleep	Poor balance/coordination
Easily distracted	Poor concentration
Fatigue	Ringing in ears
Feel "in a fog"	Sadness
Feel "slowed down"	Seeing stars
Headache	Sensitivity to light
Inappropriate emotions	Sensitivity to noise
Irritability	Sleep disturbance
Loss of consciousness	Vacant stare/glassy-eyed
Loss of orientation	Vomiting
Memory problems	

Reference

Guskiewicz KM, Bruce SL, Cantu RC, Ferrara MS, Kelly JP, McCrea M, Putukian M, VcLeod TC. National Athletic Trainers' Association Position Statement: Management of Sports Related Concussion. *J Athl Train.* 2004; 39: 280–297.

List Additional Signs/Symptoms of concussion that you have seen:

Range of Motion

Students should know the typical values of range of motion for the following joints. They should also know how to assess each joint and be able to explain the difficulties of interpreting the results of ROM tests. In many joints the observed motion comes from multiple articulations. Because of this combination of movements, it is difficult to assign a number to explain a range of motion. Therefore, students must not only know typical values for range of motion but also the limitations of using these values to describe joint movement.

	Typical Values			Typical Values
Toes			**Trunk**	
Flexion	35°–45°		Flexion	Touch floor
Extension	75°–85°		Extension	30°
			Lateral Flexion	Hand to knee
Ankle			Rotation	90°
Inversion	20°			
Eversion	5°		**Neck**	
Plantar Flexion	50°		Flexion	Chin to chest
Dorsiflexion	20°		Extension	Look to ceiling
			Lateral Flexion	45°
Knee			Rotation	90°
Flexion	135°–145°			
Extension	0°–(−10°)		**Elbow**	
			Flexion	145°–155°
Hip			Extension	0°–(−5°)
Flexion	120°–130°			
Extension	10°–20°		**Shoulder**	
Abduction	45°		Flexion	170°–180°
Adduction	30°		Extension	50°–60°
Internal Rotation	45°		Abduction	170°–180°
External Rotation	50°		Adduction	30°–40°

(continues)

(continued)

	Typical Values		Typical Values
Shoulder		**Finger**	
Internal Rotation	80°–90°	MP Joints	
External Rotation	90°–100°	Flexion	90°
Horizontal Abduction	135°	Extension	20°
Horizontal Adduction	60°	DIP & PIP	
Forearm		Flexion	90°
Pronation	90°	Extension	0°
Supination	90°	**Thumb**	
Wrist		Flexion at MP	60°–70°
Flexion	80°–90°	Extension	0°
Extension	75°–85°	Abduction	70°–80°
Radial Deviation	20°	Adduction	5°–10°
Ulnar Deviation	35°	Opposition	touch fingers

CHAPTER 23

Abbreviations – People, Policy, and Organizations

Athletic Trainers should be familiar with each of the abbreviations below. Knowing the abbreviations and the purpose of each organization will assist in written and oral communication with other professionals.

AAFP – American Academy of Family Physicians

ACI – Approved Clinical Instructor

ACSM – American College of Sports Medicine

ADA – Americans with Disabilities Act

AED – Automated External Defibrillator

AHA – American Heart Association

AMA – American Medical Association

AOSS – American Orthopedic Society for Sports

APTA – American Physical Therapy Association

ARC – American Red Cross

ATC – Certified Athletic Trainer

ATEJ – Athletic Training Education Journal

BA – Bachelor of Arts

BOC – Board of Certification

BS – Bachelor of Science

CAATE – Commission on Accreditation of Athletic Training Education

CARF – Commission on Accreditation of Rehabilitation Facilities

CDC – Centers for Disease Control and Prevention

CEU – Continuing Education Units

CI – Clinical Instructor

CIE – Clinical Instructor Educator

CMS – Centers for Medicare and Medicaid Services

CPR – Cardiopulmonary Resuscitation

CPT – Current Procedural Terminology (treatment codes)

CSCS – Certified Strength and Conditioning Specialist

DA – Doctor of Arts

DC – Doctor of Chiropractic

DDS – Doctor of Dental Surgery

DO – Doctor of Osteopathy

DPE – Doctor of Physical Education

DPM – Doctor of Podiatric Medicine

DPT – Doctor of Physical Therapy

EC – Education Council

EdD – Doctor of Education

EDS – Education Specialist

EEOC – Equal Employment Opportunity Commission

EMS – Emergency Medical Service

EMT – Emergency Medical Technician

EMTP – Emergency Medical Technician - Paramedic

FACSM – Fellow American College of Sports Medicine

FDA – Food and Drug Administration

FERPA – Family Educational Rights Privacy Act

FLSA – Fair Labor Standards Act

FMLA – Family Medical Leave Act

HIPAA – Health Insurance Portability and Account-ability Act

HMO – Health Maintenance Organization

ICD-9-CM – International Classification of Diseases-9th Ed-Clinical Modification (diagnostic codes)

IOC – International Olympic Committee

JAT – Journal of Athletic Training

LPN – Licensed Practical Nurse

MA – Master of Arts

MEd – Master of Education

MD – Medical Doctor

MS – Master of Science

NAIA – National Association of Intercollegiate Athletics

NATA – National Athletic Trainers' Association

NATABOC – See BOC

NATAPAC – National Athletic Trainers' Association Political Action Committee

NCAA – National Collegiate Athletic Association

NP – Nurse Practitioner

NREMT – National Registry of Emergency Medical Technicians

NSCA – National Strength and Conditioning Association

OSHA – Occupational Safety and Health Administration

OT – Occupational Therapist

PA – Physician's Assistant

PhD – Doctor of Philosophy

PPO – Preferred Provider Organization

PT – Physical Therapist

PTA – Physical Therapy Assistant

RD – Registered Dietitian

RDA – Recommended Daily Allowance

REF – Research and Education Foundation

RN – Registered Nurse

USDA – United States Department of Agriculture

USOC – United States Olympic Committee

Medical Conditions

Athletic Trainers should be able to explain medical conditions to colleagues in professional language. They should also be able to explain the etiology and treatment of a variety of medical conditions to patients.

Abscess
Achilles tendonitis
Amenorrhea
Amnesia
Anaphylaxis
Anemia
Anesocoria
Aneurysm
Angina
Ankylosis
Anorexia
Anteversion of the hip
Anxiety
Aortic regurgitation
Apnea
Apophysitis
Appendicitis
Apraxia
Arrythmogenic right ventricular dysplasia
Arthritis
Asthma

Bacteremia
Bennett fracture
Bipolar disorder
Bradycardia
Bronchitis
Bulimia
Bursitis
Carbuncle
Carpal tunnel syndrome
Cataract
Cellulitis
Cerebral aneurysm
Cerebral palsy
Cerebrovascular accident (CVA)
Cervical cancer
Cervical dislocation
Cervical fracture
Chickenpox
Chondromalacia patella
Chronic fatigue syndrome

Chronic obstructive pulmonary disease (COPD)
Claudication
Colitis
Colles' fracture
Commotio cordis
Compartment syndrome
Concussion
Congestive heart failure
Conjunctivitis
Constipation
Contact dermatitis
Convulsions
Coronary artery disease
Corneal abrasion
Corneal laceration
Crackles
Croup
Cryptorchidism
Cushing's syndrome

Deep vein thrombosis (DVT)
Dental caries
Depression
Dermatitis
Detached retina
Deviated septum
Diabetes
Diarrhea
Dislocation
Dysmenorrhea
Dysphagia
Dysuria
Ectopic pregnancy
Eczema
Encephalitis
Endocarditis
Endometriosis
Epicondylitis
Epididymitis
Epidural hematoma
Epilepsy
Epistaxis

Epstein-Barr virus

Erythema

Esophgeal reflux

Exercise-induced bronchospasm (EIB)

Extensor tendon avulsion

Facet syndrome

Fibromyalgia

Flexor tendon avulsion

Folliculitis

Fracture

Frostbite

Ganglion

Gastritis

Gastroenteritis

Gastroesophageal reflux

Gastrointestinal infection

Genital warts

Genu recurvatum

Genu valgus

Genu varus

Gingivitis

Glaucoma

Gout

Gynecomastia

Heart murmur

Heat exhaustion

Heat stroke

Heat syncope

Hematoma

Hematuria

Hemolysis

Hemophilia

Hemorrhoids

Hemothorax

Hepatitis

Hepatitis B

Hepatomegaly

Herpes simplex

Herpes zoster

Hip dislocation

HIV/AIDS

Hives

Human papilloma virus

Hydrocele

Hyperemia

Hypertension

Hyperthermia

Hyperthyroidism

Hypertrophic cardiomyopathy

Hyperventilation

Hyphema

Hypotension

Hypothermia

Hypothyroidism

Iliotibial band friction syndrome

Impacted cerumen

Impetigo

Indigestion

Infection

Inflammatory bowel disease

Influenza

Intracranial hemorrhage

Irritable bowel syndrome

Jaundice

Jaw (TMJ) dislocation

Kidney stones

Kyphosis

Laryngitis

Legg-Calve-Perthe's disease

Leukemia

Liver contusion

Lordosis

Lower respiratory infection (LRI)

Lupus

Lyme disease

Lymphagitis

Malaise

Mandible fracture

Marfan syndrome

Maxilla fracture

Measles

Melanoma

Meningitis

Meniscus tears

Metacarpal fracture

Methicillin-resistant Staphylococcus Aureus (MRSA)

Migraine headache

Mitral valve prolapse

Mononucleosis (Mono)

Monochordism

Multiple sclerosis

Mumps

Myocardial infarction

Myocarditis

Myositis

Nasal fracture

Nerve root compression

Nerve root stretch

Neuroma

Nystagmus

Oligomenorrhea

Orbital fracture (blowout fracture)

Osgood-Schlatter disease

Osteitis pubis

Osteochondritis dissecans

Osteomyelitis

Osteoporosis

Otitis externa

Otitis interna

Otitis media

Ovarian cancer

Pancreatitis

Patella femoral pain syndrome

Pelvic inflammatory disease

Pelvic obliquity

Peptic ulcer

Pericarditis

Peripheral embolism

Peroneal nerve contusion

Pes cavus

Pes planus

Pharyngitis

Pinna hematoma (Cauliflower ear)

Piriformis syndrome

Pleurisy

Pneumonia

Pneumothorax

Popliteal cyst

Post concussion syndrome

Post grade amnesia

Psoriasis

Pubalgia

Pulmonary embolism

Raynaud's disease/ phenomenon

Reflex sympathetic dystrophy

Retrograde amnesia

Retroversion of the hip

Rhabdomyolysis

Rhinitis

Ringworm

Rubella

Rupture

Ruptured tympanic membrane

Sacroiliac dysfunction

Salter-Harris fractures (I - VI)

Schmorel's node

Scoliosis

Seasonal affective disorder (SAD)

Second impact
    syndrome

Seizure

Segond Fracture

Sepsis

Sexually transmitted
    diseases

Sickle cell anemia

Sinusitis

Slipped capital
    femoral epiphysis

Spina bifida

Splenomegaly

Spondylolisthesis

Spondylolysis

Sprain

Staph infection

Stenosis

Strain

Stress fracture

Stridor

Stye

Subdural hematoma

Subluxation

Syncope

Syphilis

Tendinitis

Tension
    pneumothorax

Testicular
    cancer

Tetanus

Tibial torsion

Tinea capitus

Tinea cruris

Tinea pedis

Tinea versicolor

Tinnitus

Tonsillitis

Tooth avulsion

Tooth fracture

Tuberculosis

Ulcer

Undescended
    testicle

Upper respiratory
    infection

Urinary tract
    infection

Varicella

Varicocele

Viral diseases

Vertigo

Wheezes

Winged
    scapulae

Wolf-Parkinson-
    White syndrome

CHAPTER 25

Physiological Values

Athletic Trainers are often in a position to explain or interpret physiological values for their patients. Below is a listing of many physiological variables and their values. Where the variable is affected by age (e.g., body composition) values are reported for a young (20-year-old) population. The reader should know that these values are presented as guidelines for understanding typical physiological values. These numbers are not absolute values for making clinical decisions.

HEART FUNCTIONS

	Heart Rate (beats/minute)
Resting – Adult	60–80
Resting – Endurance Trained	< 60 can be as low as 30
Maximal	Max HR = 220 minus age
Cardiac Output	4.8–6.4 L/min
Stroke Volume	60–80 ml up to 180 ml during exercise
Ejection Fraction	60%

PHYSICAL ACTIVITY INTENSITY COMPARED TO PERCENT MAXIMUM HEART RATE

Intensity	% Maximum HR
Very Light	< 50
Light	50–63
Moderate	64–76
Hard	77–93
Very Hard	> 94
Maximal	100

BLOOD PRESSURE

Classification	Systolic/Diastolic mmHg
Normal	< 120/80
Prehypertension	120–139/ 80–89
Hypertension	
Stage 1	140–159/90–99
Stage 2	> 160/100

BLOOD COMPOSITION

		% of Total Blood
Plasma	% of Plasma	**55**
Water	90	
Plasma Proteins	7	
Other	3	
Formed Elements	% of Formed Elements	**45**
Red Blood Cells	99	
White Blood Cells and Platelets	1	
Total Blood Volume	5L (up to 7L in highly trained individuals)	**100**

BLOOD ANALYSIS

Variable	Men	Neutral	Women
Hemoglobin (g/dL)	13.5–17.5		11.5–15.5
Hematocrit (%)*	40–52		36–58
Red Cell Count ($\times 10^{12}$/L)	4.5–6.5		3.9–5.6
White Cell Count ($\times 10^{9}$/L)		4–11	
Platelet Count ($\times 10^{9}$/L)		150–450	
Fasting Glucose (mg/dL)		60–109	
Blood Urea Nitrogen mg/dL		4–24	
Creatinine (mg/dL)		.3–1.4	
Uric Acid (mg/dL)	4.0–8.9		2.3–7.8
Sodium (mEq/L)		135–150	
Potassium (mEq/L)		3.5–5.5	
Chloride (mEq/L)		98–110	

(*continues*)

(continued)

Variable	Men	Neutral	Women
Calcium (mg/dL)		8.5–10.5	
Phosphorus (mg/dL)		2.5–4.5	
Total Protein (g/dL)		6.0–8.5	
Albumin (g/dL)		3.0–5.5	
Iron (mg/dL)	40–190		35–180
Bilirubin (mg/dL)		< 1.5	
pH		Rest = 7.4 (neutral) Intense Exercise ~ 6.5 (acidic)	

* Hematocrit – Ratio of formed elements in the blood to total blood volume.

BLOOD GLUCOSE IN RELATION TO DIABETES

Test	GlucoseLevel mg/dL	Assessment
0 hour fast	> 200 & polyuria, polydipsia	Diabetes
2 hour fast	100–140	Normal
2 hour fast	> 200	Diabetes
8 hour fast	60–80	Normal
8 hour fast	100–125	Prediabetes
8 hour fast	> 126	Diabetes
Random	< 126	Normal
Random	< 60	Hypoglycemia
Random	> 180	Hyperglycemia

CIRCULATION DISTRIBUTION

Organ	At Rest %	Activity %
Brain	15	3–4
Heart	4–5	4–5
Digestive System	20–25	3–5
Kidneys	20	2–4
Bone	3–5	.5–1
Skin	4–5	Trace
Skeletal Muscle	15–20	80–85

OXYGEN CONCENTRATION IN THE BODY

Rest	O_2 Content in Arteries	20 ml/100ml
Rest	O_2 Content in Veins	14 ml/100ml
Rest	a-vO_2 difference	6 ml/100ml
Activity	a-vO_2 difference	15 ml/100 ml

LUNG VOLUMES/RATES

Function	Definition	Amount
Vital Capacity	Amount of air that can be expelled after maximal inspiration.	6 L
Residual Volume	Amount of air that cannot be removed from the lungs.	1.2 L
Tidal Volume	Amount of air breathed in and out during normal respiration	.5 L
Inspiratory Reserve	Maximum inspiration at the end of tidal volume	2.5 L
Expiratory Reserve	Maximum expiration at the end of tidal expiration	1 L
Ventilation	Amount of air exchanged in 1 minute	
Rest		6 L/min
Strenuous Exercise		175 L/min
Respiratory Rate		
Rest		12 b/min
Exercise		40– 50 b/min
V02 Max	Maximal amount of O_2 a person can use	
Untrained		40 ml/kg/min
Aerobically Trained		75 ml/kg/min

MET = Metabolic Equivalent = the amount of oxygen your body consumes during rest relative to body weight. 1 MET = 3.5 ml/kg/min

BODY MASS INDEX (BMI)

Classification	kg/m^2
Underweight	< 18.5
Normal	18.5–24.9
Overweight	25–29.9
Obese	
I	30–34.9
II	35–39.9
III	> 40

PERCENT BODY FAT

Classification	Men	Women
Essential	3–5	8–12
Low/Athletic	6–7	13–20
Recommended	8–19	21–32
Overfat	20–24	33 –38
Obese	> 25	> 39

WAIST TO HIP RATIO

Category	Men	Women
Excellent	≤ 0.85	≤ 0.72
Good	0.86–0.92	0.73–0.78
Fair	0.93–1.0	0.79–0.96
Poor	> 1.0	>0.96

WATER

Water constitutes about 55% of our body weight.

Weight loss of 2–4% can adversely affect performance.

A loss of 9–12% of total body weight can be fatal.

BONE MINERAL DENSITY

T Score	Assessment
(+1) – (−.99)	Normal
(−1) – (−2.5)	Below Normal (bone thinning)
> (− 2.5)	Osteoporosis

CHOLESTEROL & TRIGLYCERIDE LEVELS

LDL	
< 100	Optimal
100–129	Near optimal
130–159	Borderline High
160–189	High
> 190	Very high

(*continues*)

(*continued*)

HDL

< 40	Low
> 60	High

Total Cholesterol

< 200	Desirable
200–239	Borderline High
> 240	High

Triglycerides

< 150	Normal
150–199	Borderline high
200–499	High
> 500	Very high

URINALYSIS

Component	Normal
Color	Light Yellow
Specific gravity	1.003–1.030
RBC	< 5 HPF High Powered Field
WBC	< 5 HPF High Powered Field
Protein	Negative
Glucose	Negative
Ketones	Negative
Nitrites	Negative

REFLEX SCORES

Score	Reflex Activity
0	Absent
1	Trace
2	Normal
3	Slightly hyperactive
4	Hyperactive with clonus (i.e., repetitive vibratory movements)
5	Sustained clonus

RISK OF DEVELOPING CARDIOVASCULAR DISEASE

Risk Factor	Very Low	Low	Moderate	High	Very High
Blood Pressure (mm/Hg)					
Systolic	<110	120	130–140	156–160	> 170
Diastolic	< 70	76	82–88	94–100	> 106
Total Cholesterol (mg/dl)	<180	<200	220–240	260–280	> 300
Triglycerides (mg/dl)	< 50	< 100	> 130	> 200	> 300
Glucose (mg/dl)	< 80	90	100–110	120–130	> 140
Body Fat %					
Men	12	16	25	30	> 35
Women	16	20	30	35	> 40
Body Mass Index	< 25	25–30	30–40	> 40	

MUSCLE GLYCOGEN STORES

Level	mmol/kg
Low	50
Normal	100
High	200

BODY TEMPERATURE

Fahrenheit	Assessment	Centigrade
94	Hypothermia	34.5
98.6	Normal	37
102	Low Grade Fever	39
104	High Grade Fever	40

ATMOSPHERE

Concentration (%)	Oxygen (O_2)	20.93
	Carbon Monoxide (CO_2)	.03
	Nitrogen (N_2)	79.04
Pressure (mmHg)	Sea Level	760
	10 Meters below sea level	1500
	High Altitude	250

STRENGTH AND ENDURANCE

Exercise	Normal – Good
Bench Press	
Men	1.1–1.5 1 RM/Body Weight
Women	.7–.9 1 RM/Body Weight
Leg Press	
Men	1.9–2.3 1 RM/Body Weight
Women	1.5–1.8 1 RM/Body Weight
Push Ups to Failure	
Men	27–40
Women	20–32
Partial Curl Ups to Failure	
Men	27–75
Women	27–70
YMCA Sit and Reach	
Men	18–22 inches
Women	20–24 inches

References

American College of Sports Medicine. *ACSM's Guidelines for Exercise Testing and Prescription* 7th Ed. Lippincott Williams & Wilkins. 2006.

Cuppett M, Walsh KM. *General Medical Conditions in the Athlete.* Elsevier Mosby. 2005.

Fahey TD, Insel PM, Roth WT. *Fit and Well: Core Concepts and Labs in Physical Fitness and Wellness* 7th Ed. McGraw Hill. 2007.

McArdle WD, Katch IK, Katch VL. *Exercise Physiology: Energy, Nutrition and Human Performance* 5th Ed. Lippincott Williams & Wilkins. 2001.

Powers SK, Howley ET. *Exercise Physiology: Theory and Application to Fitness and Performance.* 6th Ed. McGraw Hill. 2007.

Wilmore JH, Costill DL. *Physiology of Sport and Exercise* 2nd Ed. Human Kinetics. 1999.

CHAPTER 26

Muscles–Illustrations

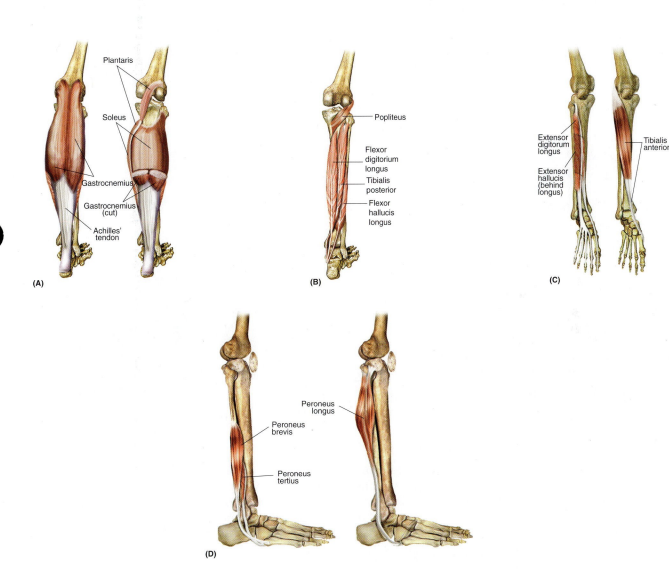

Figure 26.1 Muscles of the Foot and Ankle (A) Posterior; gastrocnemius, soleus, plantaris (B) Posterior Deep; tibialis posterior, flexor digitorum, flexor hallucis, popliteus (C) Anterior; tibialis anterior, extensor digitorum, extensor hallucis (D) Lateral; peroneus tertius, peroneus longus, peroneus brevis

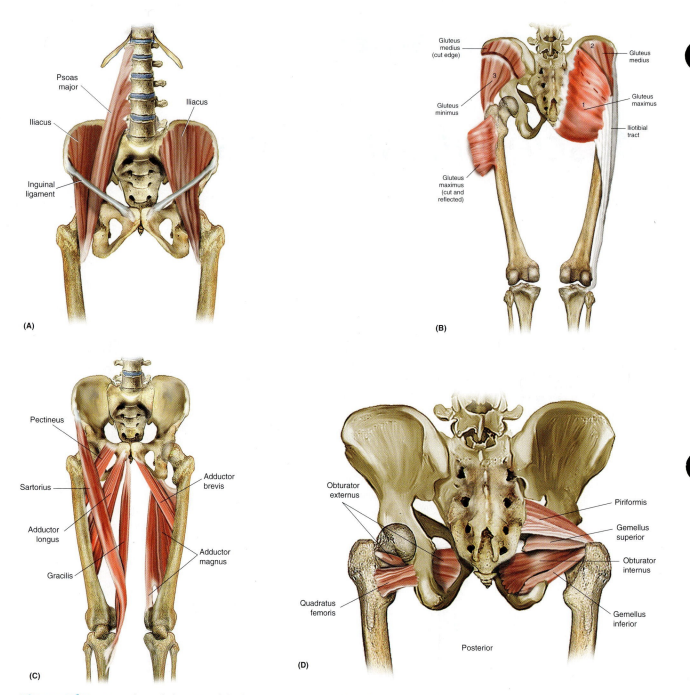

Figure 26.2 Muscles of the Hip (A) Iliacus and psoas (B) gluteus maximus, gluteus minimus, gluteus medius (C) pectineus, adductor magnus, adductor longus, adductor brevis, gracilis, sartorius (C) obtrator externus and internus, gemellus superior and inferior, quadratus femoris, piriformis (Note: The tensor fascia lata is not shown. See Figure 26-1A for the semitendinous and semimembranosus.)

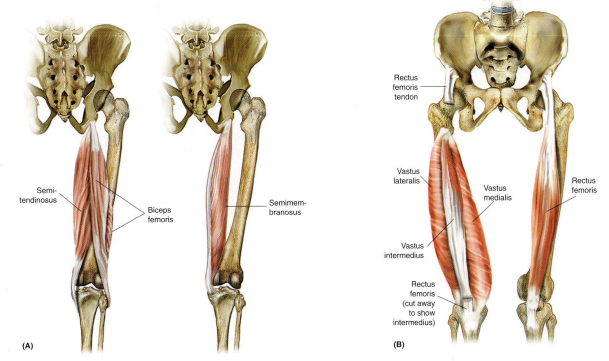

Figure 26.3 Muscles of the Knee (A) Posterior; semitendinosus, biceps femoris, semimembranosus (B) Anterior; vastus lateralis, vastus medialis, vastus intermedius, rectus femoris (Note: for position of popliteus see Figure 26-1B.)

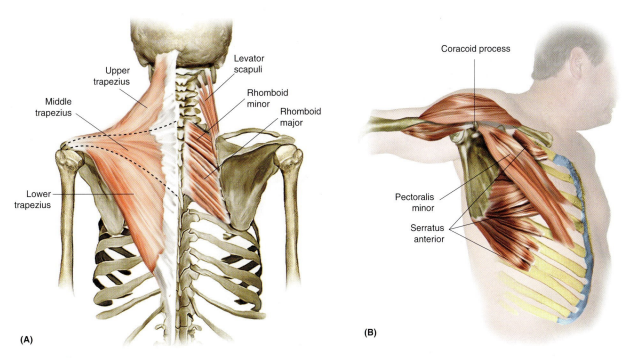

Figure 26.4 Muscles of the Scapula (A) upper trapezius, middle trapezius, lower trapezius, levator scapuli, rhomboid major and minor (B) pectoralis minor and serratus anterior

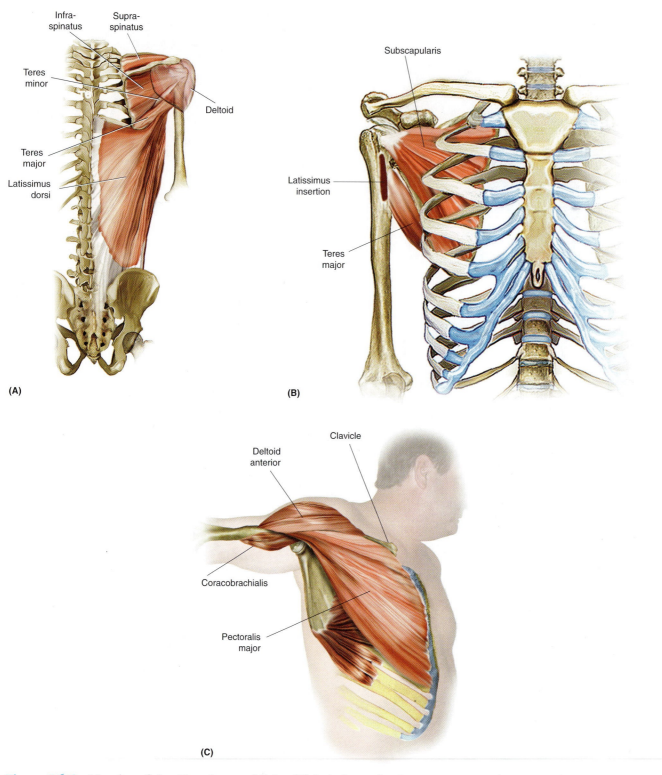

Figure 26.5 Muscles of the Glenohumeral Joint (A) latissimus dorsi, teres major and minor, infraspinatus, supraspinatus, deltoid (B) subscapularis (C) pectoralis major, deltoid, coracobrachialis (Note: the biceps brachii is shown in Figure 26-6A)

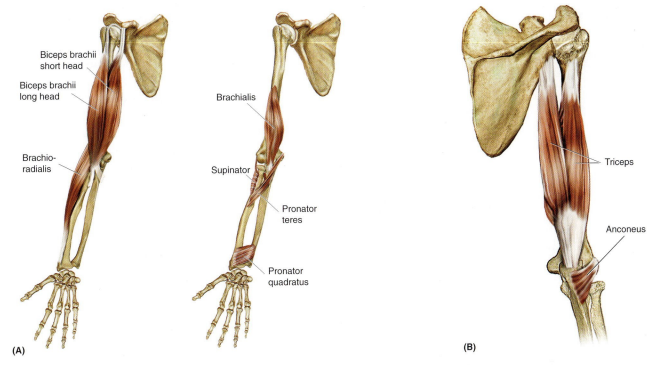

Figure 26.6 Muscles of the elbow (A) biceps brachii, brachioradialis, brachialis, supinator, pronator teres, pronator quadratus (B) triceps and aconeus

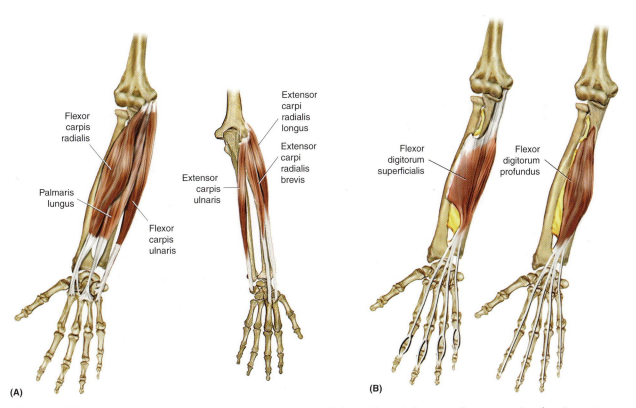

Figure 26.7 Muscles of the Wrist (A) flexor carpis radialis, Palmaris longus, flexor carpis ulnaris, extensor carpis ulnaris, extensor carpi radialis longus, extensor carpi radialis brevis (B) flexor digitorum superficialis and flexor digitorum profundus (Note: flexor pollicis longus is shown in Figure 26-8C)

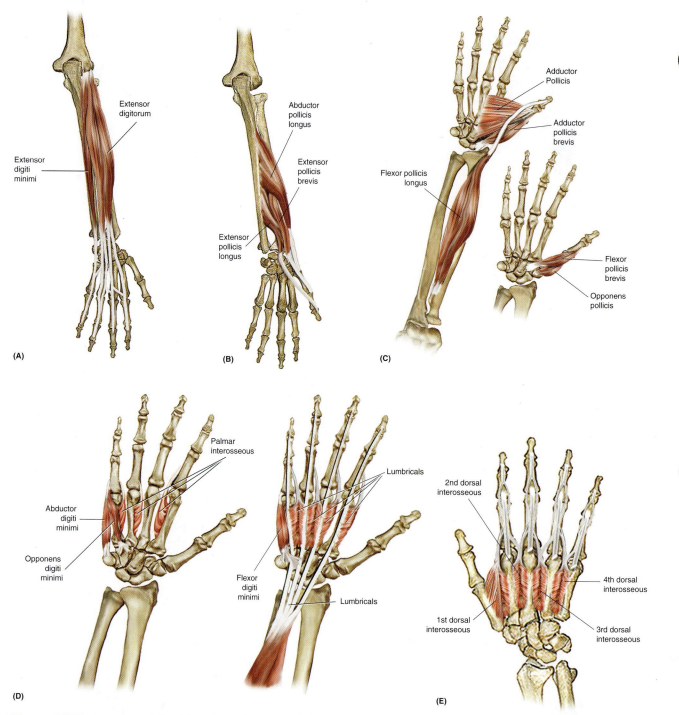

Figure 26.8 Muscles of the Thumb and Fingers (A) extensor digitorum and extensor digiti minimi (B) abductor pollicis longus, extensor pollicis brevis, and extensor pollicis longus (C) adductor pollicis, abductor pollicis brevis, flexor pollicis longus, flexor pollicis revis, and opponens pollicis (D) palmar interosseous, abductor digiti minimi, oponens digit minimi, flexor digiti minimi, lumbricals (E) dorsal interossi (Note: the extensor indicis is not shown)

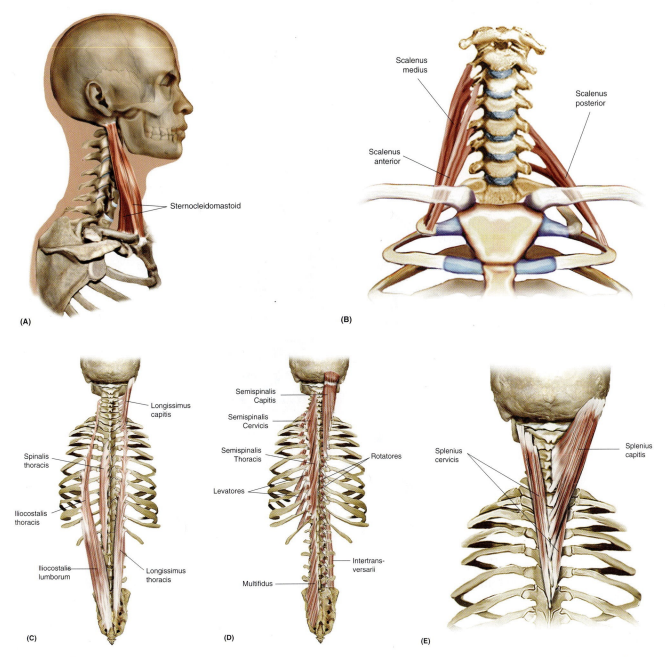

Figure 26.9 Muscles of the Back and Neck (A) Sternocleidomastoid (B) Scalenus anterior, scalenus medius, and scalenus posterior (C) Longissimus capitus, longissimus thoracis, spinalis thoracis, iliocostalis thoracis, and iliocostalis lumborum (D) semispinalis capitis, semispinalis cervicis, semispinalis thoracis, levatores (E) splenius cervicis and splenius capitis

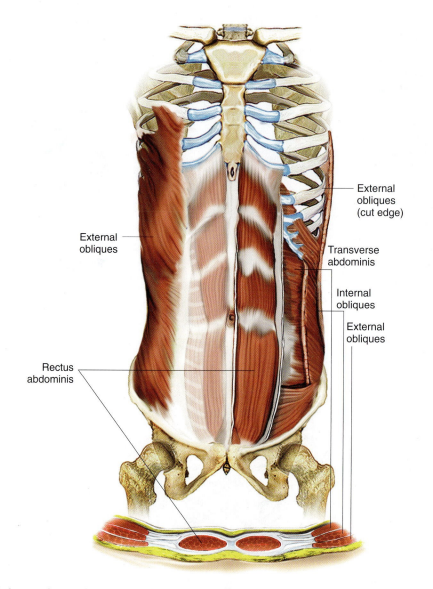

Figure 26.10 Abdominal muscles: rectus abdominis, external obliques, internal obliques, and transverse abdominis

External
obliques
(cut edge)

Transverse
abdominis

Internal
obliques

External
obliques

External
obliques

Rectus
abdominis

CHAPTER 27

Concept Maps of the Body Systems

Athletic Trainers continuously apply their knowledge of anatomy and physiology to assess and recondition patients. This chapter is included to remind students of the integral relationship of form and function of the body systems. (From Rizzo *Fundamentals of Anatomy and Physiology* 2nd Ed, Thomson Publishing, 2006)

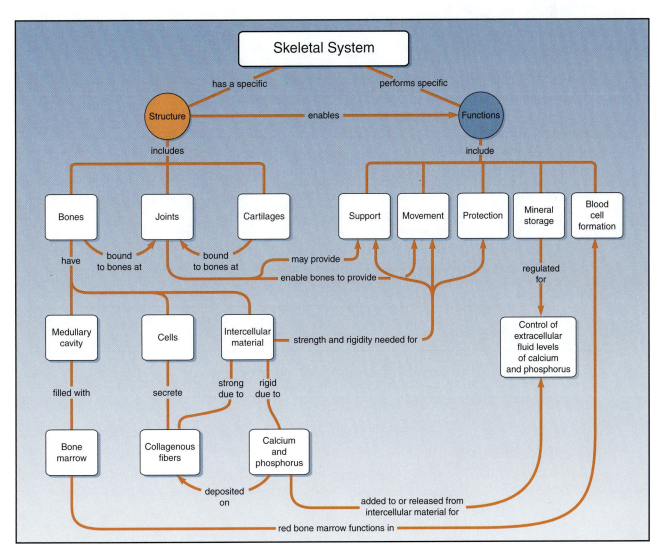

Figure 27.1   Skeletal System Concept Map

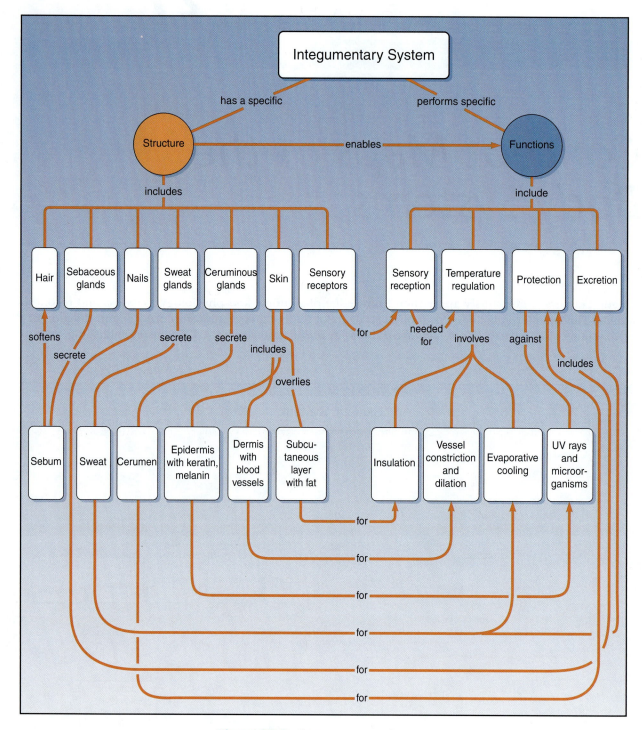

Figure 27.2 Integumentary System

232

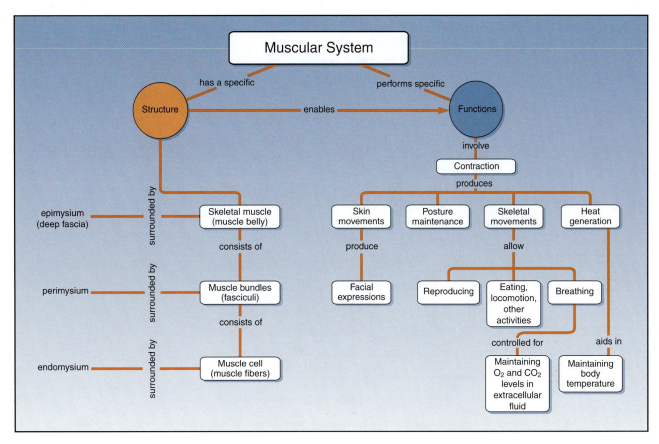

Figure 27.3 Muscular System Concept Map

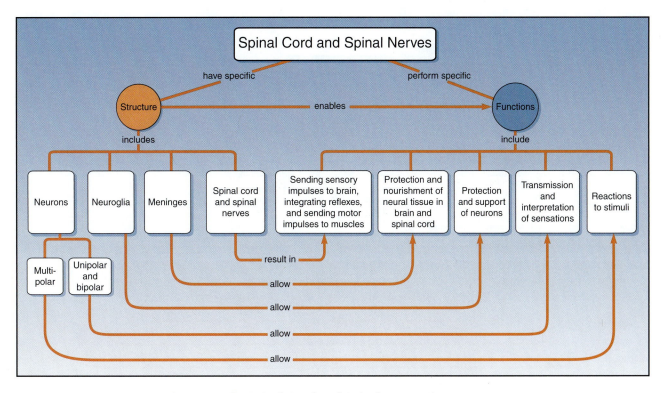

Figure 27.4 Spinal Cord and Spinal Nerves Concept Map

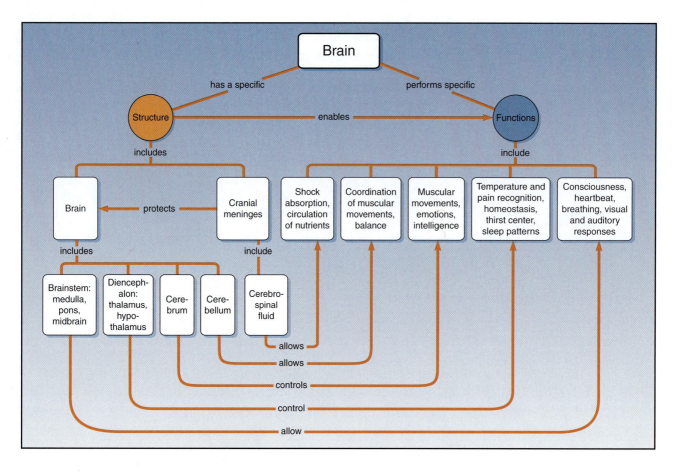

Figure 27.5 Brain Concept Map

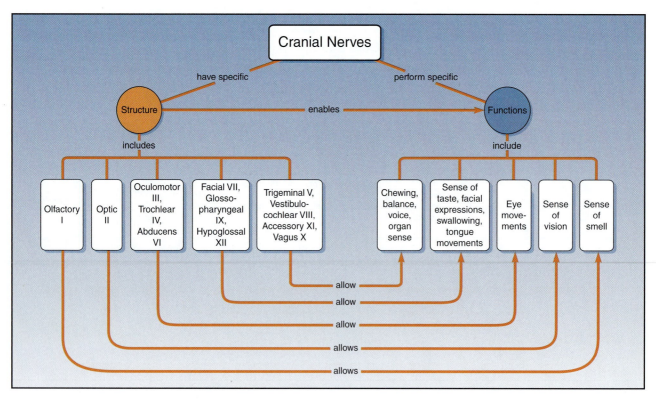

Figure 27.6 Cranial Nerves Concept Map

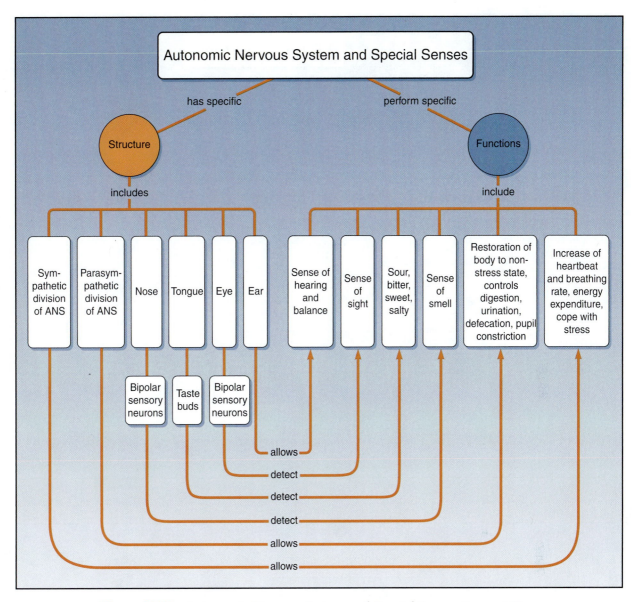

Figure 27.7   Autonomic Nervous System and Special Senses Concept Map

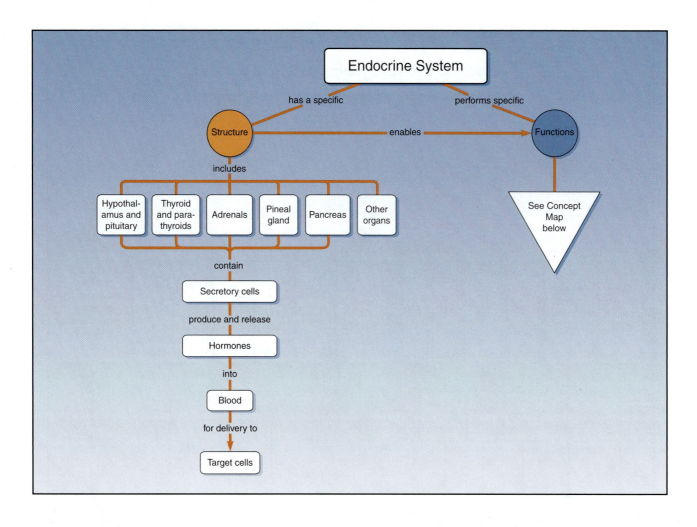

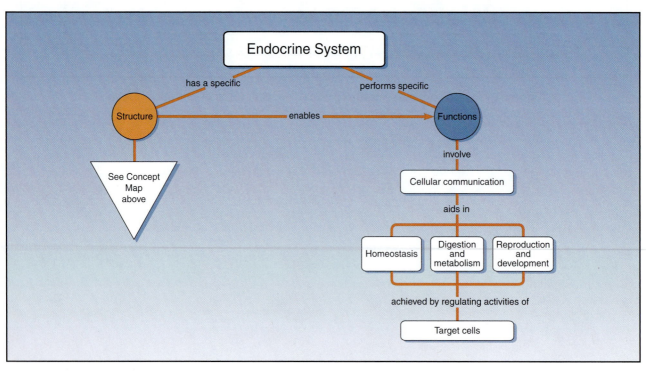

Figure 27.8 Endocrine System Concept Map

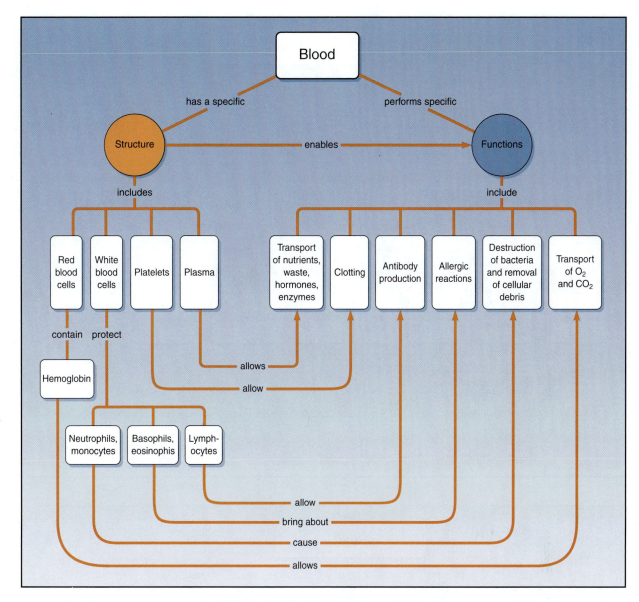

Figure 27.9   Blood Concept Map

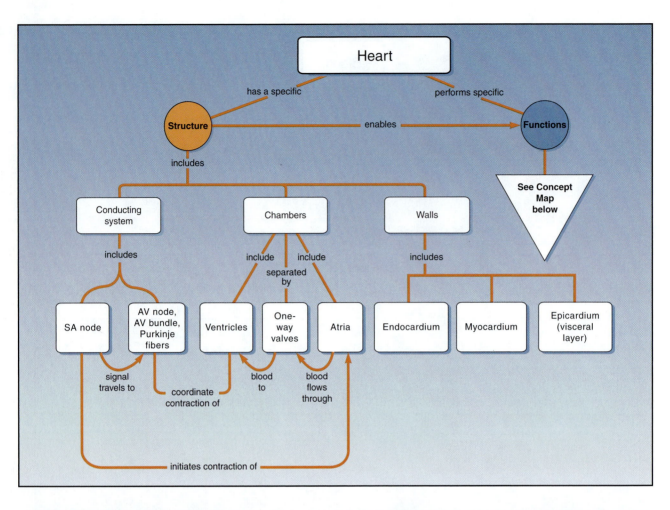

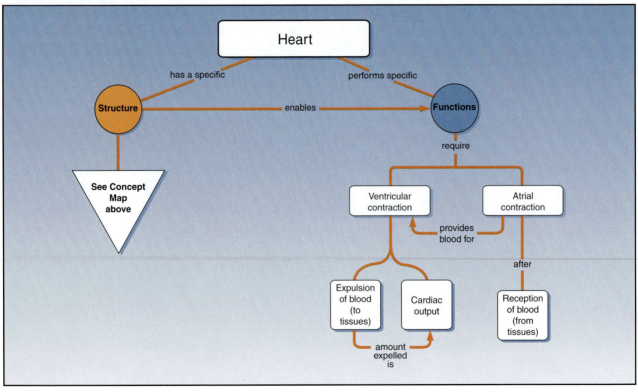

Figure 27.10   Heart Concept Map

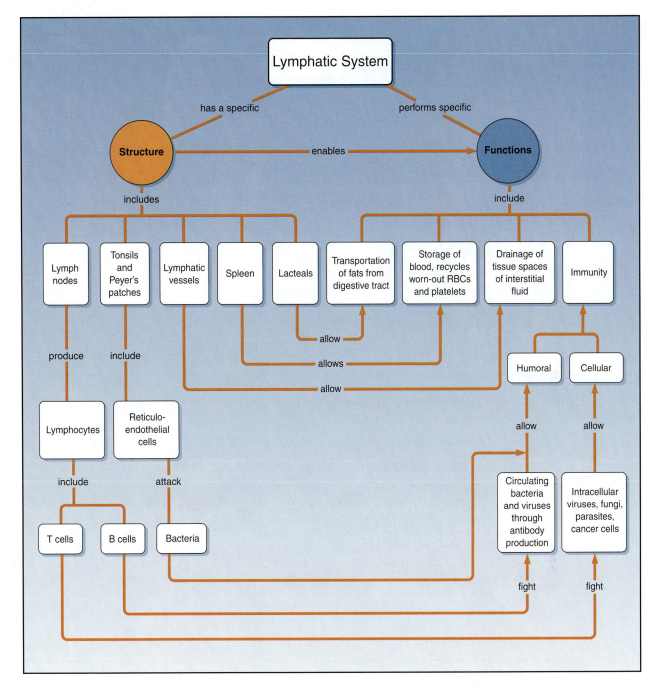

Figure 27.11 Lymphatic System Concept Map

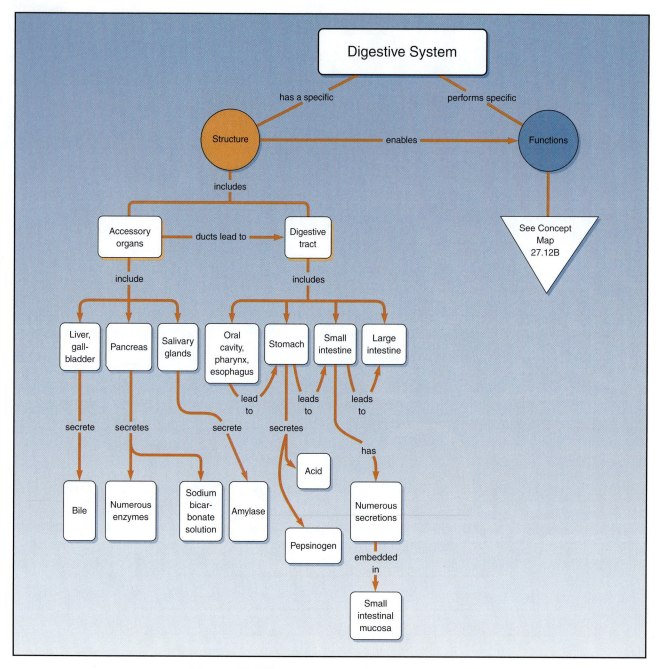

Figure 27.12A Digestive System Concept Map

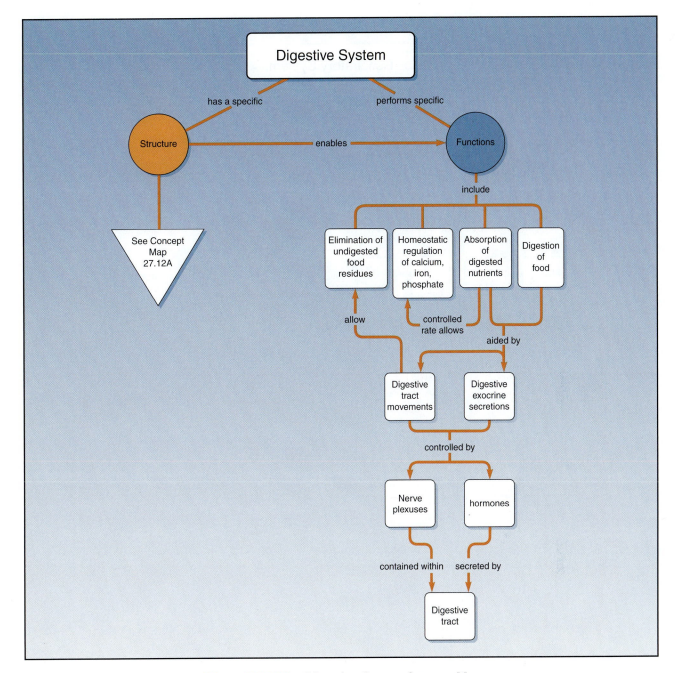

Figure 27.12B   Digestive System Concept Map

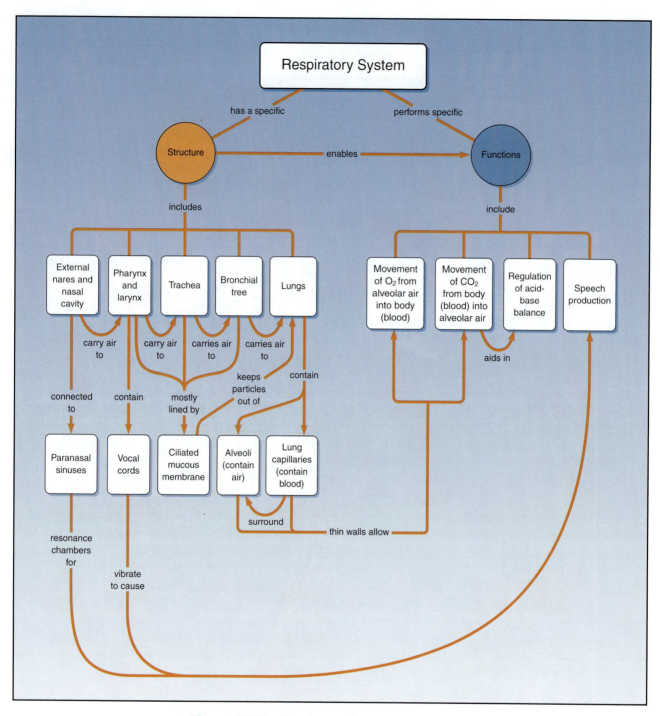

Figure 27.13 Respiratory System Concept Map

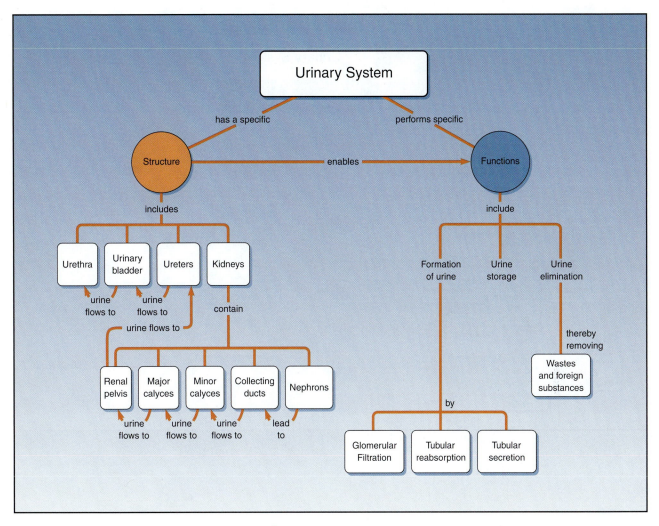

Figure 27.14A   Urinary System Concept Map

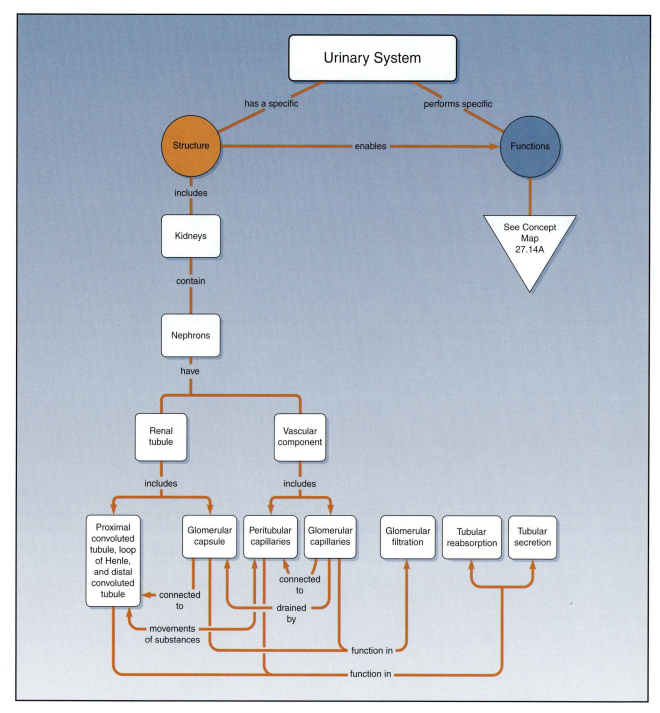

Figure 27.14B Urinary System Concept Map

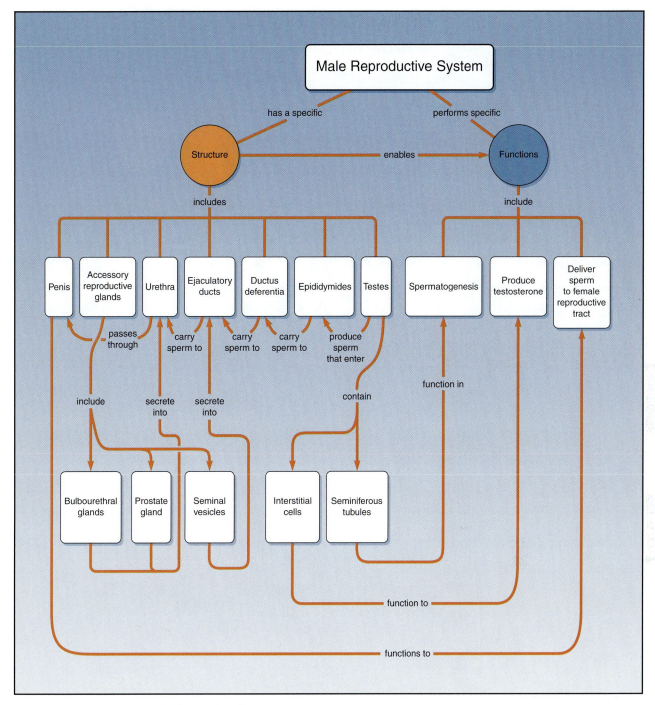

Figure 27.15   Male Reproductive System Concept Map

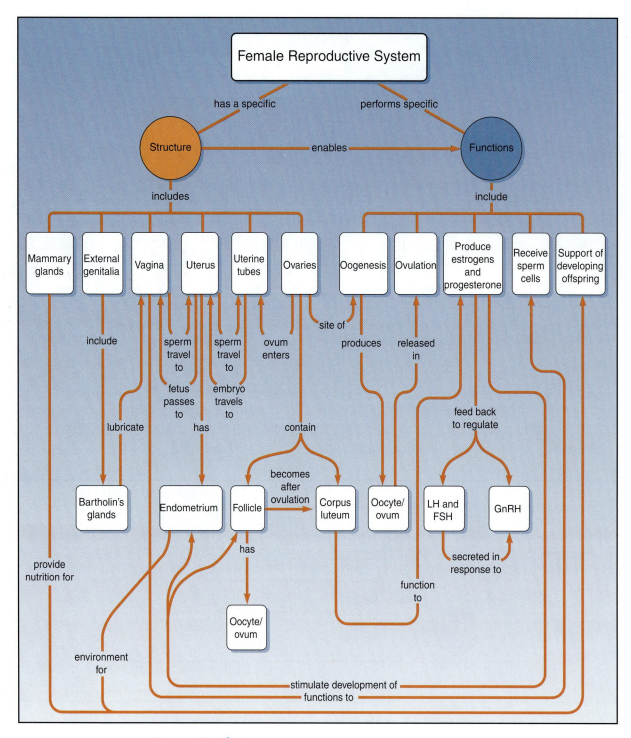

Figure 27.16 Female Reproductive System Concept Map

Clinical Skills Scoring Rubrics

This section contains scoring rubrics for the skills presented in chapters 4–16. Each skill set has two rubrics. One rubric is for the novice student. The other rubric is for the advanced student. The novice student should be focused on performing the skill properly. Therefore the rubric is based on the quality of the skill performance. The advanced student should be focused on making decisions about what skills are necessary for treating a patient and how the results of those skills should be interpreted. The advanced student rubric criteria are therefore not a listing of the skills but rather a higher level of interpretation of skills.

Assessment of the novice student should be in a controlled environment in which the student is given a specific skill to perform. Assessment of the advanced student should take place in a real or simulated situation. In a real situation the students should include or exclude appropriate skills. The instructor should ask the student questions to determine if the student has a thorough understanding of the situation. See the advanced student rubric for the type of knowledge/skill a student should possess in order to meet the advanced student requirements. An additional way of determining if a student is advanced is to present a situation that requires multiple skill sets and thus multiple rubrics. For example, a neck injury may require an athletic trainer to assess vital signs, level of consciousness, and neurological integrity. A competent athletic trainer can include all pertinent skill sets, exclude counterproductive skills, and explain her decisions to others.

VITAL SIGNS

Novice Student

Assessment Date _____   Student _____   CI/ACI _____

The novice student should be able to:

1. assess all vital signs correctly
2. identify expected/normal patient response
3. identify unexpected/pathological patient response

Skill	Unsatisfactory 0	Acceptable 1	Exceptional 2
Airway/Breathing			
Circulation			
Bleeding			
Skin Temp and Color			
Blood Pressure			
Pulse Rate and Rhythm			
Pupils			
Additional Skills			

Total Score _____

Explanation of Unsatisfactory marks:

Explanation of Exceptional marks:

VITAL SIGNS

Advanced Student

Assessment Date _____   Student _____   CI/ACI _____

The advanced athletic training student must be able to:

1. satisfy all novice criteria by performing skill correctly
2. explain the **how** and **why** for each assessment
3. make choices about what to include/exclude from evaluation
4. interpret test results in the context of the situation at hand
5. list possible pathologies/outcomes as they are progressing through the differential diagnosis
6. answer questions from patients, health care providers, coaches, parents, etc.

BREATHING, CIRCULATION, BLEEDING, SKIN, BLOOD PRESSURE, PULSE, PUPILS

Skill	Unsatisfactory 0	Acceptable 1	Exceptional 2
Performs skills correctly			
Explains How?			
Explains Why?			
Makes choices about what to include/exclude from evaluation			
Interprets test results in the context of the situation at hand			
Lists possible pathologies/outcomes of findings			
Answers questions well			
Additional Criteria			

Total Score _____

Explanation of Unsatisfactory marks:

Explanation of Exceptional marks:

BODY COMPOSITION

Assessment Date _____   Student _____   CI/ACI _____

The novice student should be able to:

1. perform all tests correctly (e.g., hand placement, pressure, etc.)
2. perform steps in the proper order
3. calculate properly

Skill	Unsatisfactory 0	Acceptable 1	Exceptional 2
BMI			
Skin Fold			

Total Score _____

Explanation of Unsatisfactory marks:

Explanation of Exceptional marks:

BODY COMPOSITION

Assessment Date _____   Student _____   CI/ACI _____

The advanced athletic training student must be able to:

1. satisfy all novice criteria by performing skill correctly
2. explain the **how** and **why** for each different body composition assessment
3. interpret results in the context of the situation at hand
4. answer questions from patients, health care providers, coaches, parents, etc.

BMI, BODY COMPOSITION

Skill	Unsatisfactory 0	Acceptable 1	Exceptional 2
Performs skills correctly			
Explains How?			
Explains Why?			
Interprets findings correctly			
Answers questions well			
Additional Criteria			

Total Score _____

Explanation of Unsatisfactory marks:

Explanation of Exceptional marks:

BASELINE MEASUREMENTS

Novice Student

Assessment Date _____   Student _____   CI/ACI _____

The novice student should be able to:

1. perform all components of the measurement correctly (e.g., goniometer placement, pressure, etc.)
2. perform steps in a logical order
3. identify expected/normal patient response
4. identify unexpected/pathological patient response

Skill	Unsatisfactory 0	Acceptable 1	Exceptional 2
Limb Girth			
Limb Length			
Vision			
Posture			
Flexibility			
Strength			

Total Score _____

Explanation of Unsatisfactory marks:

Explanation of Exceptional marks:

BASELINE MEASUREMENTS

Advanced Student

Assessment Date _____   Student _____   CI/ACI _____

The advanced student must be able to:

1. satisfy all novice criteria by performing skill correctly
2. explain the **how** and **why** for each different baseline assessment
3. interpret results in the context of the situation at hand
4. answer questions from patients, health care providers, coaches, parents, etc.

LIMB, VISION, POSTURE, FLEXIBILITY, STRENGTH

Skill	Unsatisfactory 0	Acceptable 1	Exceptional 2
Performs skills correctly			
Explains How?			
Explains Why?			
Interprets findings correctly			
Answers questions correctly			
Additional Criteria			

Total Score _____

Explanation of Unsatisfactory marks:

Explanation of Exceptional marks:

SPLINTING

Assessment Date _____   Student _____   CI/ACI _____

The novice student should be able to:

1. apply all splints correctly
2. check to ensure the splint is secure
3. check circulation before and after splint is applied
4. identify expected/normal patient response
5. identify unexpected/pathological patient response

Skill	Unsatisfactory 0	Acceptable 1	Exceptional 2
Ankle			
Knee			
Hip			
Shoulder			
Elbow			
Wrist			
Finger			
Additional Skills			

Total Score _____

Explanation of Unsatisfactory marks:

Explanation of Exceptional marks:

SPLINTING

Assessment Date _____ Student _____ CI/ACI _____

The advanced student must be able to:

1. satisfy all novice criteria by performing skill correctly
2. explain the **how** and **why** for each different splint
3. modify splint as needed to match the situation
4. interpret results in the context of the situation at hand
5. answer questions from patients, health care providers, coaches, parents, etc.

ANKLE, KNEE, HIP, SHOULDER, ELBOW, WRIST, FINGER

Skill	Unsatisfactory 0	Acceptable 1	Exceptional 2
Performs skills correctly			
Explains How?			
Explains Why?			
Modifies as needed			
Interprets findings correctly			
Answers questions correctly			
Additional Criteria			

Total Score _____

Explanation of Unsatisfactory marks:

Explanation of Exceptional marks:

EQUIPMENT FITTING

Novice Student

Assessment Date _____   Student _____   CI/ACI _____

The novice student should be able to:

1. pre-measure as is appropriate for the equipment
2. fit equipment to the athlete
3. check to ensure proper fit
4. adjust equipment as needed

Skill	Unsatisfactory 0	Acceptable 1	Exceptional 2
Equipment Fitting			
Helmet			
Shoulder Pads			
Footwear			
Mouth Guard			
Knee Brace			
Ankle Brace			

Total Score _____

Explanation of Unsatisfactory marks:

Explanation of Exceptional marks:

EQUIPMENT FITTING

Assessment Date _____   Student _____   CI/ACI _____

The advanced student must be able to:

1. satisfy all novice criteria by performing skill correctly
2. explain the **how** and **why** proper fitting is important for each protective equipment
3. make a judgment about the quality of the fit
4. answer questions from patients, health care providers, coaches, parents, etc.

HELMET, SHOULDER PADS, FOOTWEAR, MOUTH GUARD, KNEE BRACE, ANKLE BRACE

Skill	Unsatisfactory 0	Acceptable 1	Exceptional 2
Performs skills correctly			
Explains How?			
Explains Why?			
Makes judgment about the quality of the fit			
Answers questions well			
Additional Criteria			

Total Score _____

Explanation of Unsatisfactory marks:

Explanation of Exceptional marks:

TAPING

Novice Student

Assessment Date _____   Student _____   CI/ACI _____

The novice student should be able to:

1. perform all taping techniques correctly
2. perform steps in the proper order
3. exhibit proper mechanics (e.g., no wrinkles)
4. identify expected/normal patient response
5. identify unexpected/pathological patient response

Skill	Unsatisfactory 0	Acceptable 1	Exceptional 2
Ankle #1			
Ankle #2			
Arch			
Lower Leg			
Toe			
Wrist			
Thumb			
Elbow			
Fingers			

Total Score _____

Explanation of Unsatisfactory marks:

Explanation of Exceptional marks:

TAPING

Assessment Date _____   Student _____   CI/ACI _____

The advanced athletic training student must be able to:

1. satisfy all novice criteria by performing skill correctly
2. explain the **how** and **why** for each taping procedure
3. modify taping procedures in the context of the situation at hand
4. answer questions from patients, health care providers, coaches, parents, etc.

ANKLE, ARCH, LOWER LEG, TOE, WRIST, THUMB, ELBOW, FINGERS

Skill	Unsatisfactory 0	Acceptable 1	Exceptional 2
Performs skills correctly			
Explains How?			
Explains Why?			
Modifies as needed			
Answers questions Well			
Additional Criteria			

Total Score _____

Explanation of Unsatisfactory marks:

Explanation of Exceptional marks:

ELASTIC WRAPS

Novice Student

Assessment Date _____   Student _____   CI/ACI _____

The novice student should be able to:

1. perform all procedures correctly
2. exhibit proper mechanics (e.g., pressure from wrap)
4. identify expected/normal patient response
5. identify unexpected/pathological patient response

Skill	Unsatisfactory 0	Acceptable 1	Exceptional 2
Ankle			
Ankle – Cloth wrap			
Knee			
Hamstrings			
Quadriceps			
Hip – Flexors			
Hip – Adductors			
Shoulder			
Elbow			

Total Score _____

Explanation of Unsatisfactory marks:

Explanation of Exceptional marks:

ELASTIC WRAPS

Assessment Date _____   Student _____   CI/ACI _____

The advanced athletic training student must be able to:

1. satisfy all novice criteria by performing skill correctly
2. explain the **how** and **why** for each procedure
3. modify wrap procedures in the context of the situation at hand
4. answer questions from patients, health care providers, coaches, parents, etc.

ANKLE, KNEE, HAMSTRING, QUAD, HIP, SHOULDER, ELBOW

Skill	Unsatisfactory 0	Acceptable 1	Exceptional 2
Performs skills correctly			
Explains How?			
Explains Why?			
Modifies appropriately			
Answers questions correctly			
Additional Criteria			

Total Score _____

Explanation of Unsatisfactory marks:

Explanation of Exceptional marks:

HYDRATION ASSESSMENT

Novice Student

Assessment Date _____ Student _____ CI/ACI _____

The novice student should be able to:

1. perform all procedures correctly
2. identify expected/normal patient response
3. identify unexpected/pathological patient response

Skill	Unsatisfactory 0	Acceptable 1	Exceptional 2
Sling Psychrometer			
Urine Analysis			
Refractometer			

Total Score _____

Explanation of Unsatisfactory marks:

Explanation of Exceptional marks:

HYDRATION ASSESSMENT

Assessment Date _____   Student _____   CI/ACI _____

The advanced athletic training student must be able to:

1. satisfy all novice criteria by performing assessment correctly
2. explain the **how** and **why** for each assessment
3. interpret test results in the context of the situation at hand
5. list possible pathologies/outcomes as they are progressing through the differential diagnosis
6. answer questions from patients, health care providers, coaches, parents, etc.

SLING PSYCHROMETER, URINALYSIS, REFRACTOMETER

Skill	Unsatisfactory 0	Acceptable 1	Exceptional 2
Performs skills correctly			
Explains How?			
Explains Why?			
Interprets test results in the context of the situation at hand			
Lists possible pathologies/outcomes of findings			
Answers questions correctly			
Additional Criteria			

Total Score _____

Explanation of Unsatisfactory marks:

Explanation of Exceptional marks:

SYSTEMIC PATHOLOGY ASSESSMENT SKILLS

Assessment Date _____   Student _____   CI/ACI _____

The novice student should be able to:

1. perform all tests correctly
2. perform steps in the proper order
3. exhibit proper mechanics (e.g., hand placement, pressure, etc.)
4. identify expected/normal patient response
5. identify unexpected/pathological patient response

Skill	Unsatisfactory 0	Acceptable 1	Exceptional 2
Otoscope			
Ophthalmoscope			
Stethoscope			
Heart sounds			
Lung sounds			
Bowel sounds			

Total Score _____

Explanation of Unsatisfactory marks:

Explanation of Exceptional marks:

SYSTEMIC PATHOLOGY ASSESSMENT SKILLS

Advanced Student

Assessment Date _____   Student _____   CI/ACI _____

The advanced athletic training student must be able to:

1. satisfy all novice criteria by performing skill correctly
2. explain the **how** and **why** for each assessment
3. make choices about what to include/exclude from evaluation
4. interpret test results in the context of the situation at hand
5. list possible pathologies/outcomes as they are progressing through the differential diagnosis
6. answer questions from patients, health care providers, coaches, parents, etc.

OTOSCOPE, OPHTHALMOSCOPE, STETHOSCOPE

Skill	Unsatisfactory 0	Acceptable 1	Exceptional 2
Performs skills correctly			
Explains How?			
Explains Why?			
Makes choices about what to include/exclude from evaluation			
Interprets test results in the context of the situation at hand			
Lists possible pathologies/outcomes of findings			
Answers questions correctly			
Additional Criteria			

Total Score _____

Explanation of Unsatisfactory marks:

Explanation of Exceptional marks:

FOOT, ANKLE, AND LEG EVALUATION

Assessment Date _____   Student _____   CI/ACI _____

The novice student should be able to:

1. perform all tests correctly
2. perform steps in the proper order
3. exhibit proper mechanics (e.g., hand placement, pressure, etc.)
4. identify expected/normal patient response
5. identify unexpected/pathological patient response

Skill	Unsatisfactory 0	Acceptable 1	Exceptional 2
History/Subjective			
Observation			
Static Posture			
Dynamic Posture			
Deformity			
Palpation			
Soft Tissue			
Bones and Landmarks			
ROM (Act and Pass)			
Toe – Flx and Ext			
Inversion			
Eversion			
Plantar Flexion			
Dorsiflexion			
Strength			
Toe Flx and Ext			
Inversion			
Eversion			

Skill	Unsatisfactory 0	Acceptable 1	Exceptional 2
Plantar Flexion			
Dorsiflexion			
Special Tests			
Lat (ATF, CF, PTF)			
Med (Deltoid)			
Tendon			
Tib Fib Joint			
Great Toe MP			
Rule out fracture			
Circ and Neurological			
Skin Temp and Color			
Dermatomes			
Myotomes			
Reflexes			
Pulse			
Functional Activities			

Total Score _____

Explanation of Unsatisfactory marks:

Explanation of Exceptional marks:

FOOT, ANKLE, AND LEG EVALUATION

Advanced Student

Assessment Date _____   Student _____   CI/ACI _____

The advanced athletic training student must be able to:

1. satisfy all novice criteria by performing skill correctly
2. explain the **how** and **why** for each assessment
3. make choices about what to include/exclude from evaluation
4. interpret test results in the context of the situation at hand
5. list possible pathologies/outcomes as they are progressing through the differential diagnosis
6. answer questions from patients, health care providers, coaches, parents, etc.

FOOT, ANKLE, LEG – HISTORY, OBSERVATION, ROM, STRENGTH, SPECIAL, CIRCULATION, FUNCTIONAL

Skill	Unsatisfactory 0	Acceptable 1	Exceptional 2
Performs skills correctly			
Explains How?			
Explains Why?			
Makes choices about what to include/exclude from evaluation			
Interprets test results in the context of the situation at hand			
Lists possible pathologies/outcomes of findings			
Answers questions correctly			
Additional Criteria			

Total Score _____

Explanation of Unsatisfactory marks:

Explanation of Exceptional marks:

KNEE AND THIGH EVALUATION

Novice Student

Assessment Date _____   Student _____   CI/ACI _____

The novice student should be able to:

1. perform all tests correctly
2. perform steps in the proper order
3. exhibit proper mechanics (e.g., hand placement, pressure etc)
4. identify expected/normal patient response
5. identify unexpected/pathological patient response

Skill	Unsatisfactory 0	Acceptable 1	Exceptional 2
History/Subjective			
Observation			
Static Posture			
Dynamic Posture			
Deformity			
Palpation			
Soft Tissue			
Bones and Landmarks			
ROM (Act and Pass)			
Flexion			
Extension			
Patella Mobility			
Strength			
Flexion			
Extension			
Special Tests			
ACL			
PCL			

(continues)

(*continued*)

Skill	Unsatisfactory 0	Acceptable 1	Exceptional 2
MCL			
LCL			
Meniscus			
Iliotibial Band			
Patella tests			
Femur (Stress Fx)			
Rule out fracture			
Circ and Neurological			
Skin Temp and Color			
Dermatomes			
Myotomes			
Reflexes			
Pulse			
Functional Activities			

Total Score _____

Explanation of Unsatisfactory marks:

Explanation of Exceptional marks:

KNEE AND THIGH EVALUATION

Advanced Student

Assessment Date _____   Student _____   CI/ACI _____

The advanced athletic training student must be able to:

1. satisfy all novice criteria by performing skill correctly
2. explain the **how** and **why** for each assessment
3. make choices about what to include/exclude from evaluation
4. interpret test results in the context of the situation at hand
5. list possible pathologies/outcomes as they are progressing through the differential diagnosis
6. answer questions from patients, health care providers, coaches, parents, etc.

KNEE, THIGH – HISTORY, OBSERVATION, ROM, STRENGTH, SPECIAL, CIRCULATION, FUNCTIONAL

Skill	Unsatisfactory 0	Acceptable 1	Exceptional 2
Performs skills correctly			
Explains How?			
Explains Why?			
Makes choices about what to include/exclude from evaluation			
Interprets test results in the context of the situation at hand			
Lists possible pathologies/outcomes of findings			
Answers questions correctly			
Additional Criteria			

Total Score _____

Explanation of Unsatisfactory marks:

Explanation of Exceptional marks:

HIP EVALUATION

Assessment Date _____   Student _____   CI/ACI _____

The novice student should be able to:

1. perform all tests correctly
2. perform steps in the proper order
3. exhibit proper mechanics (e.g., hand placement, pressure, etc.)
4. identify expected/normal patient response
5. identify unexpected/pathological patient response

Skill	Unsatisfactory 0	Acceptable 1	Exceptional 2
History/Subjective			
Observation			
Static Posture			
Dynamic Posture			
Deformity			
Palpation			
Soft Tissue			
Bones and Landmarks			
ROM (Act and Pass)			
Flexion			
Extension			
Abduction			
Adduction			
Rotation			
Strength			
Flexion			
Extension			

Skill	Unsatisfactory 0	Acceptable 1	Exceptional 2
Abduction			
Adduction			
Circumduction			
Special Tests			
Pubofemoral Lig			
Iliofemoral Lig			
Ischiofemoral Lig			
Acetabulum			
Pubic Symphysis			
Rule out fracture			
Circ and Neurological			
Skin Temp and Color			
Dermatomes			
Myotomes			
Reflexes			
Pulse			
Functional Activities			

Total Score _____

Explanation of Unsatisfactory marks:

Explanation of Exceptional marks:

HIP EVALUATION

Advanced Student

Assessment Date _____   Student _____   CI/ACI _____

The advanced athletic training student must be able to:

1. satisfy all novice criteria by performing skill correctly
2. explain the **how** and **why** for each assessment
3. make choices about what to include/exclude from evaluation
4. interpret test results in the context of the situation at hand
5. list possible pathologies/outcomes as they are progressing through the differential diagnosis
6. answer questions from patients, health care providers, coaches, parents, etc.

HIP – HISTORY, OBSERVATION, ROM, STRENGTH, SPECIAL, CIRCULATION, FUNCTIONAL

Skill	Unsatisfactory 0	Acceptable 1	Exceptional 2
Performs skills correctly			
Explains How?			
Explains Why?			
Makes choices about what to include/exclude from evaluation			
Interprets test results in the context of the situation at hand			
Lists possible pathologies/outcomes of findings			
Answers questions correctly			
Additional Criteria			

Total Score _____

Explanation of Unsatisfactory marks:

Explanation of Exceptional marks:

BACK AND NECK EVALUATION

Novice Student

Assessment Date _____   Student _____   CI/ACI _____

The novice student should be able to:

1. perform all tests correctly
2. perform steps in the proper order
3. exhibit proper mechanics (e.g., hand placement, pressure, etc.)
4. identify expected/normal patient response
5. identify unexpected/pathological patient response

Skill	Unsatisfactory 0	Acceptable 1	Exceptional 2
History/Subjective			
Observation			
Static Posture			
Dynamic Posture			
Deformity			
Palpation			
Soft Tissue			
Bones and Landmarks			
ROM (Act and Pass)			
Flexion			
Extension			
Lateral Flexion			
Rotation			
Strength			
Flexion			
Extension			
Lateral Flexion			
Rotation			
Limb Strength			

(continues)

(continued)

Skill	Unsatisfactory 0	Acceptable 1	Exceptional 2
Special Tests			
Sacroiliac Joint			
Facets			
Discs			
Intervert Foramen			
Rule out fracture			
Circ and Neurological			
Skin Temp and Color			
Dermatomes			
Myotomes			
Reflexes			
Pulse			
Functional Activities			

Total Score_____

Explanation of Unsatisfactory marks:

Explanation of Exceptional marks:

BACK AND NECK EVALUATION

Assessment Date _____   Student _____   CI/ACI _____

The advanced athletic training student must be able to:

1. satisfy all novice criteria by performing skill correctly
2. explain the **how** and **why** for each assessment
3. make choices about what to include/exclude from evaluation
4. interpret test results in the context of the situation at hand
5. list possible pathologies/outcomes as they are progressing through the differential diagnosis
6. answer questions from patients, health care providers, coaches, parents, etc.

BACK, NECK – HISTORY, OBSERVATION, ROM, STRENGTH, SPECIAL, CIRCULATION, FUNCTIONAL

Skill	Unsatisfactory 0	Acceptable 1	Exceptional 2
Performs skills correctly			
Explains How?			
Explains Why?			
Makes choices about what to include/exclude from evaluation			
Interprets test results in the context of the situation at hand			
Lists possible pathologies/outcomes of findings			
Answers questions correctly			
Additional Criteria			

Total Score _____

Explanation of Unsatisfactory marks:

Explanation of Exceptional marks:

SHOULDER AND ARM EVALUATION

Novice Student

Assessment Date _____   Student _____   CI/ACI _____

The novice student should be able to:

1. perform all tests correctly
2. perform steps in the proper order
3. exhibit proper mechanics (e.g., hand placement, pressure, etc.)
4. identify expected/normal patient response
5. identify unexpected/pathological patient response

Skill	Unsatisfactory 0	Acceptable 1	Exceptional 2
History/Subjective			
Observation			
Static Posture			
Dynamic Posture			
Deformity			
Palpation			
Soft Tissue			
Bones and Landmarks			
ROM (Act and Pass)			
Flexion			
Extension			
Abduction			
Adduction			
Int Rotation			
Ext Rotation			
Horizontal Abd			
Horizontal Add			

Skill	Unsatisfactory 0	Acceptable 1	Exceptional 2
Circumduction			
Scapular Movements			
Strength			
Flexion			
Extension			
Abduction			
Adduction			
Int Rotation			
Ext Rotation			
Horizontal Abd			
Horizontal Add			
Circumduction			
Scapular Movements			
Special Tests			
GH Stability			
Labrum			
Rotator Cuff			
Impingement			
Acromioclavicular Jt			
Sternoclavicular Jt			
Rule out fracture			
Circ and Neurological			
Skin Temp and Color			
Dermatomes			

(*continues*)

(continued)

Skill	Unsatisfactory 0	Acceptable 1	Exceptional 2
Myotomes			
Reflexes			
Pulse			
Functional Activities			

Total Score _____

Explanation of Unsatisfactory marks:

Explanation of Exceptional marks:

SHOULDER AND ARM EVALUATION

Advanced Student

Assessment Date _____   Student _____   CI/ACI _____

The advanced athletic training student must be able to:

1. satisfy all novice criteria by performing skill correctly
2. explain the **how** and **why** for each assessment
3. make choices about what to include/exclude from evaluation
4. interpret test results in the context of the situation at hand
5. list possible pathologies/outcomes as they are progressing through the differential diagnosis
6. answer questions from patients, health care providers, coaches, parents, etc.

SHOULDER, ARM – HISTORY, OBSERVATION, ROM, STRENGTH, SPECIAL, CIRCULATION, FUNCTIONAL

Skill	Unsatisfactory 0	Acceptable 1	Exceptional 2
Performs skills correctly			
Explains How?			
Explains Why?			
Makes choices about what to include/exclude from evaluation			
Interprets test results in the context of the situation at hand			
Lists possible pathologies/outcomes of findings			
Answers questions well			
Additional Criteria			

Total Score _____

Explanation of Unsatisfactory marks:

Explanation of Exceptional marks:

ELBOW, WRIST, AND HAND EVALUATION

Novice Student

Assessment Date _____   Student _____   CI/ACI _____

The novice student should be able to:

1. perform all tests correctly
2. perform steps in the proper order
3. exhibit proper mechanics (e.g., hand placement, pressure, etc.)
4. identify expected/normal patient response
5. identify unexpected/pathological patient response

Skill	Unsatisfactory 0	Acceptable 1	Exceptional 2
History/Subjective			
Observation			
Static Posture			
Dynamic Posture			
Deformity			
Palpation			
Soft Tissue			
Bones and Landmarks			
ROM (Act and Pass)			
Elbow Flx			
Elbow Ext			
Elbow Pro			
Elbow Sup			
Wrist Flx			
Wrist Ext			
Radial Deviation			
Ulnar Deviation			
Thumb Movements			
Finger Movements			

Skill	Unsatisfactory 0	Acceptable 1	Exceptional 2
Special Tests			
Elbow MCL			
Elbow LCL			
Annular Lig			
Med Epicondylitis			
Lat Epicondylitis			
Wrist Stability			
Wrist TFCC			
Rule out fractures			
Circ and Neurological			
Skin Temp and Color			
Dermatomes			
Myotomes			
Reflexes			
Pulse			
Functional Activities			

Total Score _____

Explanation of Unsatisfactory marks:

Explanation of Exceptional marks:

ELBOW, WRIST, AND HAND EVALUATION

Advanced Student

Assessment Date _____ Student _____ CI/ACI _____

The advanced athletic training student must be able to:

1. satisfy all novice criteria by performing skill correctly
2. explain the **how** and **why** for each assessment
3. make choices about what to include/exclude from evaluation
4. interpret test results in the context of the situation at hand
5. list possible pathologies/outcomes as they are progressing through the differential diagnosis
6. answer questions from patients, health care providers, coaches, parents, etc.

ELBOW, WRIST, HAND – HISTORY, OBSERVATION, ROM, STRENGTH, SPECIAL, CIRCULATION, FUNCTIONAL

Skill	Unsatisfactory 0	Acceptable 1	Exceptional 2
Performs skills correctly			
Explains How?			
Explains Why?			
Makes choices about what to include/exclude from evaluation			
Interprets test results in the context of the situation at hand			
Lists possible pathologies/outcomes of findings			
Answers questions correctly			
Additional Criteria			

Total Score _____

Explanation of Unsatisfactory marks:

Explanation of Exceptional marks:

HEAD AND FACE EVALUATION

Novice Student

Assessment Date _____   Student _____   CI/ACI _____

The novice student should be able to:

1. perform all tests correctly
2. perform steps in the proper order
3. exhibit proper mechanics (e.g., hand placement, pressure, etc.)
4. identify expected/normal patient response
5. identify unexpected/pathological patient response

Skill	Unsatisfactory 0	Acceptable 1	Exceptional 2
History/Subjective			
Observation			
CSF			
Deformity			
Palpation			
Deformity			
Signs/Symptoms			
LOC			
Headache			
Concentration			
Coordination			
ST Memory			
LT Memory			
Eye function			
Cranial Nerve Assessment			

(continues)

(continued)

Skill	Unsatisfactory 0	Acceptable 1	Exceptional 2
Home instructions			
Emergency Protocols			

Total Score _____

Explanation of Unsatisfactory marks:

Explanation of Exceptional marks:

HEAD AND FACE EVALUATION

Advanced Student

Assessment Date _____   Student _____   CI/ACI _____

The advanced athletic training student must be able to:

1. satisfy all novice criteria by performing skill correctly
2. explain the **how** and **why** for each assessment
3. make choices about what to include/exclude from evaluation
4. interpret test results in the context of the situation at hand
5. list possible pathologies/outcomes as they are progressing through the differential diagnosis
6. answer questions from patients, health care providers, coaches, parents, etc.

HEAD, FACE – HISTORY, OBSERVATION, PALPATION, CONCUSSION ASSESSMENT

Skill	Unsatisfactory 0	Acceptable 1	Exceptional 2
Performs skills correctly			
Explains How?			
Explains Why?			
Makes choices about what to include/exclude from evaluation			
Interprets test results in the context of the situation at hand			
Lists possible pathologies/outcomes of findings			
Answers questions correctly			
Additional Criteria			

Total Score _____

Explanation of Unsatisfactory marks:

Explanation of Exceptional marks:

MEDICAL CONDITIONS AND DISABILITIES

Novice Student

Assessment Date _____   Student _____   CI/ACI _____

The novice student should be able to:

1. perform all tests correctly
2. exhibit proper mechanics (e.g., hand placement, pressure, etc.)
3. identify expected/normal patient response
4. identify unexpected/pathological patient response

Skill	Unsatisfactory 0	Acceptable 1	Exceptional 2
Peak flow meter			
Body temperature			
Pupil reaction			
Urinalysis			
Abdominal palpation			
Liver			
Spleen			
Appendix			
Throat/Neck palpation			
Lymph nodes			

Total Score _____

Explanation of Unsatisfactory marks:

Explanation of Exceptional marks:

MEDICAL CONDITIONS AND DISABILITIES

Advanced Student

Assessment Date _____   Student _____   CI/ACI _____

The advanced athletic training student must be able to:

1. satisfy all novice criteria by performing skill correctly
2. explain the **how** and **why** for each assessment
3. make choices about what to include/exclude from evaluation
4. interpret test results in the context of the situation at hand
5. list possible pathologies/outcomes as they are progressing through the differential diagnosis
6. answer questions from patients, health care providers, coaches, parents, etc.

PEAK FLOW, BODY TEMPERATURE, PUPIL, URINALYSIS, ABDOMINAL PALPATION, NECK PALPATION

Skill	Unsatisfactory 0	Acceptable 1	Exceptional 2
Performs skills correctly			
Explains How?			
Explains Why?			
Makes choices about what to include/exclude from evaluation			
Interprets test results in the context of the situation at hand			
Lists possible pathologies/outcomes of findings			
Correctly answers questions			
Additional Criteria			

Total Score _____

Explanation of Unsatisfactory marks:

Explanation of Exceptional marks:

EMERGENCY MANAGEMENT

Novice Student

Assessment Date _____   Student _____   CI/ACI _____

The novice student should be able to:

1. perform all tasks correctly
2. perform steps in the proper order
3. exhibit proper mechanics (e.g., hand placement, pressure, etc.)
4. identify expected/normal patient response
5. identify unexpected/pathological patient response

Skill	Unsatisfactory 0	Acceptable 1	Exceptional 2
Level of Consciousness			
Rescue Breathing			
CPR			
AED			
Assess breathing status			
Assess circulation			
Assess body temperature			
Remove facemask			
Patient transport			
Control bleeding			
Clean open wound			
Dress open wound			

Total Score _____

Explanation of Unsatisfactory marks:

Explanation of Exceptional marks:

EMERGENCY MANAGEMENT

Assessment Date _____   Student _____   CI/ACI _____

The advanced athletic training student must be able to:

1. satisfy all novice criteria by performing skill correctly
2. explain the **how** and **why** for each skill
3. make choices about what to include/exclude from assessment/treatment
4. interpret test results in the context of the situation at hand
5. list possible pathologies/outcomes as they are progressing through the differential diagnosis
6. answer questions from patients, health care providers, coaches, parents, etc.

LEVEL OF CONSCIOUSNESS, RESCUE BREATHING, CPR, AED, BREATHING STATUS, CIRCULATION, BODY TEMPERATURE, FACEMASK REMOVAL, TRANSPORT, BLEEDING, OPEN WOUND

Skill	Unsatisfactory 0	Acceptable 1	Exceptional 2
Performs skills correctly			
Explains How?			
Explains Why?			
Makes choices about what to include/exclude from evaluation			
Interprets test results in the context of the situation at hand			
Lists possible pathologies/outcomes of findings			
Answers questions correctly			
Additional Criteria			

Total Score _____

Explanation of Unsatisfactory marks:

Explanation of Exceptional marks:

IMMOBILIZATION AND CRUTCH FITTING

Novice Student

Assessment Date _____   Student _____   CI/ACI _____

The novice student should be able to:

1. perform all skills correctly
2. perform steps in the proper order
3. exhibit proper mechanics (e.g., hand placement, pressure, etc.)
4. identify expected/normal patient response
5. identify unexpected/pathological patient response
6. instruct the patient on proper use of crutches

Skill	Unsatisfactory 0	Acceptable 1	Exceptional 2
Immobilize			
Ankle			
Knee			
Hip			
Shoulder			
Elbow			
Wrist/Hand			
Spine			
Crutch Fitting			

Total Score _____

Explanation of Unsatisfactory marks:

Explanation of Exceptional marks:

IMMOBILIZATION AND CRUTCH FITTING

Advanced Student

Assessment Date _____   Student _____   CI/ACI _____

The advanced athletic training student must be able to:

1. satisfy all novice criteria by performing skill correctly
2. explain the **how** and **why** for each skill
3. make choices about what to include/exclude from skill
4. interpret patient response in the context of the situation at hand
5. answer questions from patients, health care providers, coaches, parents, etc.

ANKLE, KNEE, HIP, SHOULDER, ELBOW, WRIST, SPINE, CRUTCHES

Skill	Unsatisfactory 0	Acceptable 1	Exceptional 2
Performs skills correctly			
Explains How?			
Explains Why?			
Makes choices about what to include/exclude from evaluation			
Interprets test results in the context of the situation at hand			
Lists possible pathologies/outcomes of findings			
Answers questions correctly			
Additional Criteria			

Total Score _____

Explanation of Unsatisfactory marks:

Explanation of Exceptional marks:

MODALITY APPLICATION

Novice Student

Assessment Date _____   Student _____   CI/ACI _____

The novice student should be able to:

1. perform all tasks correctly
2. perform steps in the proper order
3. exhibit proper mechanics (e.g., pad placement, sound head movement, etc.)
4. identify expected/normal patient response
5. identify unexpected/pathological patient response

Skill	Unsatisfactory 0	Acceptable 1	Exceptional 2
Infrared modality			
Cryotherapy			
Ice packs			
Ice massage			
Chemical cold packs			
Vapocoolant spray			
Ice immersion			
Thermotherapy			
Moist heat packs			
Whirlpool baths			
Paraffin baths			
Contrast Therapy			
Diathermy			
Electrical stimulation			
Direct Current			
Iontophoresis			
For pain control			

Skill	Unsatisfactory 0	Acceptable 1	Exceptional 2
For muscle contraction			
Ther ultrasound			
Pulsed US			
Continuous US			
Phonophoresis			
Traction			
Cervical			
Lumbar			
Massage			
Inter Compression			
Biofeedback			

Total Score _____

Explanation of Unsatisfactory marks:

Explanation of Exceptional marks:

MODALITY APPLICATION

Advanced Student

Assessment Date _____   Student _____   CI/ACI _____

The advanced athletic training student must be able to:

1. satisfy all novice criteria by performing skill correctly
2. explain the **how** and **why** for each modality application
3. make choices about which modalities to include/exclude from a treatment plan
4. assess the effectiveness of the modality in the context of the situation at hand
5. compare and contrast with other potential modality choices
6. answer questions from patients, health care providers, coaches, parents, etc.

INFRARED, ELECTRICAL STIMULATION, ULTRASOUND, TRACTION, MASSAGE, COMPRESSION, BIOFEEDBACK

Skill	Unsatisfactory 0	Acceptable 1	Exceptional 2
Performs skills correctly			
Explains How?			
Explains Why?			
Makes choices about which modalities to include/exclude from treatment			
Interprets test results in the context of the situation at hand			
Compares to other modality choices			
Answers questions correctly			
Additional Criteria			

Total Score _____

Explanation of Unsatisfactory marks:

Explanation of Exceptional marks:

THERAPEUTIC EXERCISE – FOOT, ANKLE, LOWER LEG

Novice Student

Assessment Date _____   Student _____   CI/ACI _____

The novice student should be able to:

1. perform all skills correctly
2. teach exercises properly
3. exhibit proper mechanics (e.g., hand placement, pressure, etc.)
4. identify expected/normal patient response

Skill	Unsatisfactory 0	Acceptable 1	Exceptional 2
Range of Motion			
Strength			
Coordination/NM control			
Functional/Sport Specific			

Total Score _____

Explanation of Unsatisfactory marks:

Explanation of Exceptional marks:

THERAPEUTIC EXERCISE – FOOT, ANKLE, LOWER LEG

Advanced Student

Assessment Date _____ Student _____ CI/ACI _____

The advanced athletic training student must be able to:

1. satisfy all novice criteria by performing skill correctly
2. explain the **how** and **why** for each exercise
3. make choices about which exercises to include/exclude from a treatment plan
4. assess the effectiveness of the exercise in the context of the situation at hand
5. compare and contrast with other potential exercise choices
6. answer questions from patients, health care providers, coaches, parents, etc.

FOOT, ANKLE, LEG – RANGE OF MOTION, STRENGTH, COORDINATION, FUNCTION

Skill	Unsatisfactory 0	Acceptable 1	Exceptional 2
Performs skills correctly			
Explains How?			
Explains Why?			
Makes choices about which exercises to include/ exclude from treatment			
Assesses the effectiveness of the exercise in the context of the situation at hand			
Compares to other exercise choices			
Answers questions correctly			
Additional Criteria			

Total Score _____

Explanation of Unsatisfactory marks:

Explanation of Exceptional marks:

THERAPEUTIC EXERCISE – KNEE AND THIGH

Novice Student

Assessment Date _____   Student _____   CI/ACI _____

The novice student should be able to:

1. perform all skills correctly
2. teach exercises properly
3. exhibit proper mechanics (e.g. hand placement, pressure, etc.)
4. identify expected/normal patient response

Skill	Unsatisfactory 0	Acceptable 1	Exceptional 2
Range of Motion			
Strength			
Coordination/NM control			
Functional/Sport Specific			

Total Score _____

Explanation of Unsatisfactory marks:

Explanation of Exceptional marks:

THERAPEUTIC EXERCISE – KNEE AND THIGH

Advanced Student

Assessment Date _____   Student _____   CI/ACI _____

The advanced athletic training student must be able to:

1. satisfy all novice criteria by performing skill correctly
2. explain the **how** and **why** for each exercise
3. make choices about which exercises to include/exclude from a treatment plan
4. assess the effectiveness of the exercise in the context of the situation at hand
5. compare and contrast with other potential exercise choices
6. answer questions from patients, health care providers, coaches, parents, etc.

KNEE, THIGH – RANGE OF MOTION, STRENGTH, COORDINATION, FUNCTION

Skill	Unsatisfactory 0	Acceptable 1	Exceptional 2
Performs skills correctly			
Explains How?			
Explains Why?			
Makes choices about which exercises to include/ exclude from treatment			
Assesses the effectiveness of the exercise in the context of the situation at hand			
Compares to other exercise choices			
Answers questions correctly			
Additional Criteria			

Total Score _____

Explanation of Unsatisfactory marks:

Explanation of Exceptional marks:

THERAPEUTIC EXERCISE - HIP

Novice Student

Assessment Date _____   Student _____   CI/ACI _____

The novice student should be able to:

1. perform all skills correctly
2. teach exercises properly
3. exhibit proper mechanics (e.g., hand placement, pressure, etc.)
4. identify expected/normal patient response

Skill	Unsatisfactory 0	Acceptable 1	Exceptional 2
Range of Motion			
Strength			
Coordination/NM control			
Functional/Sport Specific			

Total Score _____

Explanation of Unsatisfactory marks:

Explanation of Exceptional marks:

THERAPEUTIC EXERCISE – HIP   Advanced Student

Assessment Date _____   Student _____   CI/ACI _____

The advanced athletic training student must be able to:

1. satisfy all novice criteria by performing skill correctly
2. explain the **how** and **why** for each exercise
3. make choices about which exercises to include/exclude from a treatment plan
4. assess the effectiveness of the exercise in the context of the situation at hand
5. compare and contrast with other potential exercise choices
6. answer questions from patients, health care providers, coaches, parents, etc.

HIP – RANGE OF MOTION, STRENGTH, COORDINATION, FUNCTION

Skill	Unsatisfactory 0	Acceptable 1	Exceptional 2
Performs skill correctly			
Explains How?			
Explains Why?			
Makes choices about which exercises to include/ exclude from treatment			
Assesses the effectiveness of the exercise in the context of the situation at hand			
Compares to other exercise choices			
Answers questions correctly			
Additional Criteria			

Total Score _____

Explanation of Unsatisfactory marks:

Explanation of Exceptional marks:

THERAPEUTIC EXERCISE – BACK AND NECK

Novice Student

Assessment Date _____   Student _____   CI/ACI _____

The novice student should be able to:

1. perform all skills correctly
2. teach exercises properly
3. exhibit proper mechanics (e.g. hand placement, pressure, etc.)
4. identify expected/normal patient response

Skill	Unsatisfactory 0	Acceptable 1	Exceptional 2
Range of Motion			
Strength			
Coordination/NM control			
Functional/Sport Specific			

Total Score _____

Explanation of Unsatisfactory marks:

Explanation of Exceptional marks:

THERAPEUTIC EXERCISE – BACK AND NECK

Advanced Student

Assessment Date _____   Student _____   CI/ACI _____

The advanced athletic training student must be able to:

1. satisfy all novice criteria by performing skill correctly
2. explain the **how** and **why** for each exercise
3. make choices about which exercises to include/exclude from a treatment plan
4. assess the effectiveness of the exercise in the context of the situation at hand
5. compare and contrast with other potential exercise choices
6. answer questions from patients, health care providers, coaches, parents, etc.

BACK, NECK – RANGE OF MOTION, STRENGTH, COORDINATION, FUNCTION

Skill	Unsatisfactory 0	Acceptable 1	Exceptional 2
Skill performed correctly			
Explains How?			
Explains Why?			
Makes choices about which exercises to include/exclude from treatment			
Assesses the effectiveness of the exercise in the context of the situation at hand			
Compares to other exercise choices			
Answers questions correctly			
Additional Criteria			

Total Score _____

Explanation of Unsatisfactory marks:

Explanation of Exceptional marks:

THERAPEUTIC EXERCISE – SHOULDER

Novice Student

Assessment Date _____   Student _____   CI/ACI _____

The novice student should be able to:

1. perform all skills correctly
2. teach exercises properly
3. exhibit proper mechanics (e.g., hand placement, pressure, etc.)
4. identify expected/normal patient response

Skill	Unsatisfactory 0	Acceptable 1	Exceptional 2
Range of Motion			
Strength			
Coordination/NM control			
Functional/Sport Specific			

Total Score _____

Explanation of Unsatisfactory marks:

Explanation of Exceptional marks:

THERAPEUTIC EXERCISE – SHOULDER

Advanced Student

Assessment Date _____   Student _____   CI/ACI _____

The advanced athletic training student must be able to:

1. satisfy all novice criteria by performing skill correctly
2. explain the **how** and **why** for each exercise
3. make choices about which exercises to include/exclude from a treatment plan
4. assess the effectiveness of the exercise in the context of the situation at hand
5. compare and contrast with other potential exercise choices
6. answer questions from patients, health care providers, coaches, parents, etc.

SHOULDER – RANGE OF MOTION, STRENGTH, COORDINATION, FUNCTIONSKILL

Skill	Unsatisfactory 0	Acceptable 1	Exceptional 2
Performs skill correctly			
Explains How?			
Explains Why?			
Makes choices about which exercises to include/ exclude from treatment			
Assesses the effectiveness of the exercise in the context of the situation at hand			
Compares to other exercise choices			
Answers questions correctly			
Additional Criteria			

Total Score _____

Explanation of Unsatisfactory marks:

Explanation of Exceptional marks:

THERAPEUTIC EXERCISE – ARM AND ELBOW

Novice Student

Assessment Date _____   Student _____   CI/ACI _____

The novice student should be able to:

1. perform all skills correctly
2. teach exercises properly
3. exhibit proper mechanics (e.g., hand placement, pressure, etc.)
4. identify expected/normal patient response

Skill	Unsatisfactory 0	Acceptable 1	Exceptional 2
Range of Motion			
Strength			
Coordination/NM control			
Functional/Sport Specific			

Total Score _____

Explanation of Unsatisfactory marks:

Explanation of Exceptional marks:

THERAPEUTIC EXERCISE – ARM AND ELBOW

Advanced Student

Assessment Date _____   Student _____   CI/ACI _____

The advanced athletic training student must be able to:

1. satisfy all novice criteria by performing skill correctly
2. explain the **how** and **why** for each exercise
3. make choices about which exercises to include/exclude from a treatment plan
4. assess the effectiveness of the exercise in the context of the situation at hand
5. compare and contrast with other potential exercise choices
6. answer questions from patients, health care providers, coaches, parents, etc.

ARM, ELBOW – RANGE OF MOTION, STRENGTH, COORDINATION, FUNCTION

Skill	Unsatisfactory 0	Acceptable 1	Exceptional 2
Performs skills correctly			
Explains How?			
Explains Why?			
Makes choices about which exercises to include/ exclude from treatment			
Assesses the effectiveness of the exercise in the context of the situation at hand			
Compares to other exercise choices			
Answers questions correctly			
Additional Criteria			

Total Score _____

Explanation of Unsatisfactory marks:

Explanation of Exceptional marks:

THERAPEUTIC EXERCISE – WRIST AND HAND

Novice Student

Assessment Date _____   Student _____   CI/ACI _____

The novice student should be able to:

1. perform all skills correctly
2. teach exercises properly
3. exhibit proper mechanics (e.g., hand placement, pressure, etc.)
4. identify expected/normal patient response

Skill	Unsatisfactory 0	Acceptable 1	Exceptional 2
Range of Motion			
Strength			
Coordination/NM control			
Functional/Sport Specific			

Total Score _____

Explanation of Unsatisfactory marks:

Explanation of Exceptional marks:

THERAPEUTIC EXERCISE – WRIST AND HAND

Advanced Student

Assessment Date _____   Student _____   CI/ACI _____

The advanced athletic training student must be able to:

1. satisfy all novice criteria by performing skill correctly
2. explain the **how** and **why** for each exercise
3. make choices about which exercises to include/exclude from a treatment plan
4. assess the effectiveness of the exercise in the context of the situation at hand
5. compare and contrast with other potential exercise choices
6. answer questions from patients, health care providers, coaches, parents, etc.

WRIST, HAND – RANGE OF MOTION, STRENGTH, COORDINATION, FUNCTION

Skill	Unsatisfactory 0	Acceptable 1	Exceptional 2
Performs skills correctly			
Explains How?			
Explains Why?			
Makes choices about which exercises to include/ exclude from treatment			
Assesses the effectiveness of the exercise in the context of the situation at hand			
Compares to other exercise choices			
Answers questions correctly			
Additional Criteria			

Total Score _____

Explanation of Unsatisfactory marks:

Explanation of Exceptional marks:

JOINT MOBILIZATION, AQUATIC THERAPY, AND PNF

Assessment Date _____   Student _____   CI/ACI _____

The novice student should be able to:

1. perform all skills correctly
2. teach exercises properly
3. exhibit proper mechanics (e.g. hand placement, pressure, etc.)
4. identify expected/normal patient response

Skill	Unsatisfactory 0	Acceptable 1	Exceptional 2
Joint Mobilization			
Ankle			
Knee			
Hip			
Vertebrae			
Shoulder			
Elbow			
Wrist			
Fingers and Thumb			
Aquatic Therapy			
Upper Body Injuries			
Lower Body Injuries			

(continues)

(continued)

Skill	Unsatisfactory 0	Acceptable 1	Exceptional 2
PNF			
Upper Extremity – DI			
Upper Extremity – D2			
Lower Extremity – D1			
Lower Extremity – D2			

Total Score _____

Explanation of Unsatisfactory marks:

Explanation of Exceptional marks:

JOINT MOBILIZATION, AQUATIC THERAPY, AND PNF   **Advanced Student**

Assessment Date _____   Student _____   CI/ACI _____

The advanced athletic training student must be able to:

1. satisfy all novice criteria by performing skill correctly
2. explain the **how** and **why** for each exercise
3. make choices about which exercises/techniques to include/exclude from a treatment plan
4. assess the effectiveness of the exercise/technique in the context of the situation at hand
5. compare and contrast with other potential exercise choices
6. answer questions from patients, health care providers, coaches, parents, etc.

JOINT MOBILIZATION, AQUATIC THERAPY, PNF

Skill	Unsatisfactory 0	Acceptable 1	Exceptional 2
Performs skills correctly			
Explains How?			
Explains Why?			
Makes choices about which exercises/techniques to include/exclude from treatment			
Assesses the effectiveness of the technique in the context of the situation at hand			
Compares to other exercise choices			
Answers questions correctly			
Additional Criteria			

Total Score _____

Explanation of Unsatisfactory marks:

Explanation of Exceptional marks:

POWER, AGILITY, SPEED, ENDURANCE

Novice Student

Assessment Date _____   Student _____   CI/ACI _____

The novice student should be able to:

1. perform all skills correctly
2. teach exercises properly
3. exhibit proper mechanics (e.g., hand placement, pressure, etc.)
4. identify expected/normal patient response

Skill	Unsatisfactory 0	Acceptable 1	Exceptional 2
Lower Body			
Power			
Agility			
Speed			
Endurance			
Upper Body			
Power			
Agility			
Speed			
Endurance			

Total Score _____

Explanation of Unsatisfactory marks:

Explanation of Exceptional marks:

POWER, AGILITY, SPEED, ENDURANCE

Advanced Student

Assessment Date _____   Student _____   CI/ACI _____

The advanced athletic training student must be able to:

1. satisfy all novice criteria by performing skill correctly
2. explain the **how** and **why** for each exercise
3. make choices about which exercises to include/exclude from a treatment plan
4. assess the effectiveness of the exercise in the context of the situation
5. compare and contrast with other potential exercise choices
6. answer questions from patients, health care providers, coaches, parents, etc.

LOWER BODY, UPPER BODY – POWER, AGILITY, SPEED, ENDURANCE

Skill	Unsatisfactory 0	Acceptable 1	Exceptional 2
Performs skills correctly			
Explains How?			
Explains Why?			
Makes choices about which exercises to include/ exclude from treatment			
Assesses the effectiveness of the exercise in the context of the situation at hand			
Compares to other exercise choices			
Answers questions correctly			
Additional Criteria			

Total Score _____

Explanation of Unsatisfactory marks:

Explanation of Exceptional marks:

DRUG ADMINISTRATION ASSISTANCE

Assessment Date _____   Student _____   CI/ACI _____

The novice student should be able to:

1. perform all tasks correctly
2. perform steps in the proper order
3. exhibit proper mechanics (e.g. hand placement, pressure, etc.)
4. identify expected/normal patient response
5. identify unexpected/pathological patient response

Skill	Unsatisfactory 0	Acceptable 1	Exceptional 2
Administer EpiPen			
Teach proper use of asthma inhaler			
Assist with insulin injection			

Total Score _____

Explanation of Unsatisfactory marks:

Explanation of Exceptional marks:

DRUG ADMINISTRATION ASSISTANCE

Advanced Student

Assessment Date _____   Student _____   CI/ACI _____

The advanced athletic training student must be able to:

1. satisfy all novice criteria by performing skill correctly
2. explain the **how** and **why** for each assessment
3. make choices about what to include/exclude from evaluation
4. interpret test results in the context of the situation at hand
5. list possible pathologies/outcomes as they are progressing through the differential diagnosis
6. answer questions from patients, health care providers, coaches, parents, etc.

EPIPEN, INHALER, INSULIN INJECTION

Skill	Unsatisfactory 0	Acceptable 1	Exceptional 2
Performs skills correctly			
Explains How?			
Explains Why?			
Makes choices about what to include/exclude from evaluation			
Interprets test results in the context of the situation at hand			
Lists possible pathologies/outcomes of findings			
Answers questions correctly			
Additional Criteria			

Total Score _____

Explanation of Unsatisfactory marks:

Explanation of Exceptional marks:

RECORDKEEPING

Novice Student

Assessment Date _____   Student _____   CI/ACI _____

The novice student should be able to:

Perform all tasks correctly

Skill	Unsatisfactory 0	Acceptable 1	Exceptional 2
Injury report			
Progress/rehabilitation report			

Total Score _____

Explanation of Unsatisfactory marks:

Explanation of Exceptional marks:

RECORDKEEPING

Assessment Date _____   Student _____   CI/ACI _____

The advanced athletic training student must be able to:

1. satisfy all novice criteria by performing skill correctly
2. explain the **how** and **why** for each assessment
3. make choices about what to include/exclude from evaluation
4. interpret test results in the context of the situation at hand
5. list possible pathologies/outcomes as they are progressing through the differential diagnosis
6. answer questions from patients, health care providers, coaches, parents, etc.

INJURY REPORT, PROGRESS REPORT

Skill	Unsatisfactory 0	Acceptable 1	Exceptional 2
Performs skills correctly			
Explains How?			
Explains Why?			
Makes choices about what to include/exclude from evaluation			
Interprets test results in the context of the situation at hand			
Lists possible pathologies/outcomes of findings			
Answers questions correctly			
Additional Criteria			

Total Score _____

Explanation of Unsatisfactory marks:

Explanation of Exceptional marks:

Note: Page numbers in *italics* are figures.